The Clinical Practice *of* Speech-Language Pathology

Becky Sutherland Cornett
American Speech-Language-Hearing Association

Shelly S. Chabon
University of Pittsburgh

Merrill Publishing Company
A Bell & Howell Information Company
Columbus / Toronto / London / Melbourne

Published by Merrill Publishing Company
A Bell & Howell Information Company
Columbus, Ohio 43216

This book was set in Palatino.

Administrative Editor: Vicki Knight
Production Coordinator: Carol Huston Driver
Cover Designer: Jolie Muren

Library of Congress Catalog Card Number: 87-62906
International Standard Book Number: 0-675-20808-4
Printed in the United States of America
1 2 3 4 5 6 7 8 9 — 92 91 90 89 88

To our husbands and children
for their continuing tolerance and love

To our clients and their families
for their continuing trust and inspiration

Contents

Prologue

Since beginning this book, we have both relocated and changed jobs; one of us wrote a doctoral dissertation as well. Despite these changes in responsibilities, or perhaps because of them, we have maintained a growing respect and enthusiasm for the field of speech-language pathology and audiology. Although far apart in geographic area and in work situations, we share similar thoughts about the clinical practice of speech-language pathology. It is from this shared perspective that this book was written.

Our overall goal was to provide a current, realistic, practical, and comprehensive overview of professional issues basic to the clinical practice of speech-language pathology. This book is primarily intended as a text for advanced undergraduate or graduate students preparing for careers as speech-language pathologists. It may also be used as a resource book for clinical fellows or experienced clinicians seeking information about specific issues in today's health care, issues such as team approaches to treatment, trends in health-care delivery and payment systems, and quality assessment methods. Activities included at the end of each chapter are designed to enhance and extend textual presentations.

Chapters 1 and 2 contain introductory information about the profession— who we are, what we do, and where we work. Chapter 1 traces the evolution of our professional titles, roles, and qualifications and describes the professional associations and publications of interest to speech-language pathologists and audiologists. Chapter 2 examines the various settings for clinical practice, with emphasis on current trends and issues in schools, colleges and universities, private practice, and health care.

Three attitudes or orientations to clinical practice are described in chapter 3: scientific, therapeutic, and professional. In this chapter we emphasize that the practitioner must bring to the therapeutic relationship scientific principles as well as that sometimes intangible and often misunderstood quality of ''professionalism. We believe these attitudes, taken together, are essential components of high-quality clinical work.

Chapter 4 details the key clinical services of prevention, assessment, therapy, discharge planning, and consultation. It presents a general definition, primary objectives, basic strategies, and format for each type of service in the spectrum. General principles and procedures applicable to the evaluation and treatment of all communication problems are described.

The practice of clinical report writing and record keeping is addressed in chapter 5. This chapter focuses on documentation in health care and public education as well as on the many forms of professional communication. Practical descriptions and examples are provided for clinical reports, therapy plans, progress notes and progress reports, discharge summaries, referrals, and letters. In addition, case staffings and team conferences are briefly highlighted.

Chapter 6 presents introductions to the other professionals with whom speech-language pathologists commonly interact: physicians, nurses, physical therapists, occupational therapists, psychologists, social workers, and educators. It includes a discussion of multidisciplinary, interdisciplinary, and transdisciplinary team approaches to clinical practice as well as some of the problems associated with working in teams.

Chapter 7 provides an introduction to health-care financing. Overviews of both public- and private-sector health plans include information about Medicare, Medicaid, other government programs, commercial insurance companies and Blue Cross/Blue Shield plans, health maintenance organizations, preferred provider organizations, and self-insured employers. Each section includes specific information about coverage of communicative disorders and about reimbursement for speech-language pathology services.

Chapter 8 summarizes the state of the art in evaluating the quality of health care and particularly speech-language pathology and audiology services. We begin with a search for a definition of quality and progress to quality assessment and program evaluation issues. Information about utilization review and risk management is incorporated into a discussion of quality assurance programs. Quality of care in speech-language pathology and audiology is discussed within the context of the American Speech-Language-Hearing Association's standards programs, clinical accountability research and commentary, and applications of new technology and methods to quality assurance and utilization review programs in speech-language pathology and audiology.

Finally, the epilogue presents our views, as well as those of our colleagues, on the outlook for our profession in the next decade. It is certain that Dr. Patricia Cole's criteria for a "primary profession" will keep us busy for years to come.

There are many people to whom we owe our thanks. Our colleagues contributed to this book by offering information, encouraging words, and editorial assistance. We would particularly like to recognize Drs. Ernest Burgi, Stan Dublinske, Diane Eger, Carol Frattali, Audrey Holland, Jack Matthews, and Steven White. Dr. Frattali made numerous contributions to the content and format of chapter 8, particularly. University of Pittsburgh secretaries Barbara Hess and Jan Malloy transformed our scribbles and inserts into a readable and organized text. Jan was always there when we needed her, and we needed her a lot. Beth Miller, graduate student, taught us some of the joys of word processing, and Barbara Simcic offered creative ideas about the presentation of our material.

Our reviewers Mary Ellen Brandell, Central Michigan; Jo Ellyn Smith, James Madison University; Lou Echols-Chambers, University of Illinois at Urbana-Champaign; Susan Dowling, University of Houston; and Stephanie Martin, University of Oregon, provided constructive criticism and thoughtful suggestions. Our administrative editor, Vicki Knight, offered patience, support, and very sensitive advice to keep us going.

Above all, our husbands, Dr. Robert Chabon and the Reverend Ward L. Cornett III, and our children, Michael, Stephen, Andrew, and Daniel Chabon and Andrea Cornett, endured our preoccupation with this book.

We return now to our tasks and interests, fulfilled by the realization that we have contributed what we hope is a useful store of information for students and colleagues in our field. The clinical practice of speech-language pathology is an ever-evolving process for individual practitioners as well as the profession as a whole. We must be nurtured, pushed, prompted, and sometimes redirected. The focus of clinical practice is the therapeutic relationship. Like any relationship, it requires patience, compassion, understanding, and fortitude. Unlike other relationships, however, the ultimate goal is to send the client on his or her way. It is challenging, usually rewarding, and always absorbing work. We hope you think so, too.

BSC and SSC

CHAPTER ONE

The Profession of Speech-Language Pathology and Audiology

INTRODUCTION

In a recent article about career opportunities in health fields, Sarnecky (1987) described speech-language pathology and audiology as a profession that "lets you be what you want to be" (p. 3). Offering a succinct summary of the profession, she said, "If you like working with people, putting your knowledge to use and seeking answers to your questions, you will find a career in speech-language pathology or audiology to be stimulating, challenging, and rewarding" (p. 3). Sarnecky noted that as a speech-language pathologist or audiologist one can work with computers or people—the very young or very old—and in a full range of public or private employment settings. One can be a clinical service provider, an inventor, a researcher, an administrator, a teacher, or an entrepreneur, or some combination of these.

Professional Titles

A number of titles have been applied to practitioners of speech-language pathology. These titles vary in definition, connotation, origin, popularity, and/or familiarity. Among the approximately two dozen designations in use are *speech teacher*, *speech correctionist*, *speech clinician*, *speech therapist*, *speech and language therapist*, and more recently, *speech-language pathologist*. The difficulty in agreeing on a single name reflects, in part, our history and development as professionals. It also may suggest that we have demonstrated maximum adaptability to function in a number of diverse settings. Further, it demonstrates varied attempts to describe succinctly the many skills involved in becoming a speech-language pathologist.

Among the first professional titles used were *speech teacher* and *speech correctionist*. These references, now somewhat antiquated, were popular through the mid 1900s when much, if not most, of our practice occurred in public school programs and dealt with the correction of articulation, fluency, and voice problems.

By the 1960s *speech clinician* and *speech therapist* received wide, albeit transient, acceptance. These terms exemplified our increased participation in hospitals and other health-care facilities. Although the appellation *speech therapist* is the most familiar description of the scope of the profession, this title fell out of favor for a number of reasons. First, the word *speech* was viewed as too restrictive, because we are interested in and trained to manage all aspects of communication. This objection led to alternative combinations such as *speech and language therapist* or *communication therapist*. Second, there was concern that the term *therapist* suggested a professional who works under the supervision of a physician. Many practitioners argued that this title could be misleading to other professionals as well as to the general public.

In the 1970s the terms *speech pathologist* and *speech-language pathologist* became popular, with the latter receiving the endorsement of the American Speech-Language and Hearing Association (ASHA) in 1976. Despite the fact that *speech-language pathologist* is now "official," there remains some resistance to the uniform adoption of this title.

In the 1980s the suitability and universality of the title *speech-language pathologist* continues to be debated. Russell Malone, managing editor of *Asha*, the ASHA journal, observed in the comment section of the May 1986 issue that only a minority of practitioners use their professional name. In an informal survey of 280 individuals who identified themselves as "in the area of speech-language pathology" and who had contacted the Information Resource Center of ASHA, 45% used the occupational title *speech pathologist,* and 26% used the designation *speech-language pathologist* (p. 2). Other responses to the question "What is your occupation?" included speech therapist (5%), speech and language pathologist (5%), speech and language therapist (3%), speech teacher (3%), speech and language specialist (2%), speech and language clinician (1%), speech-language therapist (1%), and speech and hearing therapist (1%) (Malone, 1986, p. 2). Malone suggested that we could significantly increase awareness of our profession if speech-language pathologists would use their official titles. Similarly, Taylor (1981) reminded us that "although professionals within the field may be able to utilize various titles and understand that they all relate to the same group of individuals, the public may not be so adept" (p. 11).

Over the years our ability to adjust to so many different work settings has thus contributed both to the rapid growth of our profession and to the limited rate of acceptance of a single professional title. A challenge of the eighties is to establish goals of quality in practice and extend our services to reach more individuals in a greater variety of work settings while we strengthen our identity as speech-language pathologists, enhance our professional stature, and assert and maintain our autonomy.

This challenge is yours.

Professional Roles and Qualifications

Speech-language pathologists and audiologists are specialists in the normal development and disorders of human communication and related areas. We provide a range of services including prevention, identification, evaluation, diagnosis, treatment, teaching, counseling, and consultation. Speech-language pathologists and audiologists also engage in basic and applied research activities related to human communication and its disorders. The activities and scope of practice of the profession are variously defined. States identify the practice of speech-language pathology and audiology through licensure laws. Other definitions are included in federal laws and regulations (e.g., the Education for All Handicapped Children Act, Public Law 94–142), publications of other regulatory bodies, and in manuals of accreditation organizations such as the Joint Commission on Accreditation of Healthcare Organizations (JCAHO). The U.S. Department of Labor's *Dictionary of Occupational Titles* (1977) provides detailed definitions of the occupations listed as "audiologist" and "speech pathologist." These definitions are found in the accompanying box. The American Speech-Language-Hearing Association issued an official Scope of Practice Statement in 1987. The statement appeared in draft form in the June 1987 issue of *Asha* (p. 43). The ASHA Executive Board approved it in August 1987, and the statement was to be considered for adoption by the Legislative Council during its November 1987 meeting.

Speech-language pathologists and audiologists qualified to provide independent clinical services hold a graduate degree in speech-language pathology or audiology, and the Certificate of Clinical Competence (CCC-SLP or CCC-A) awarded by the American Speech-Language-Hearing Association. A license to practice speech-language pathology or audiology is compulsory currently in 36 states. Requirements for the Certificate of Clinical Competence encompass the following areas: general background education, required education, academic clinical practicum, the Clinical Fellowship Year, and the National Examination in Speech-Language Pathology and/or Audiology. The American Speech-Language-Hearing Association publishes a complete description of all requirements in its *Membership and Certification Handbook,* which can be obtained directly from the Certification Section of the ASHA National Office. The requirements are revised periodically.

A demographic profile of the ASHA membership (Hyman, 1987) indicates that there are about 41,000 certified speech-language pathologists and 7,250 audiologists. About 1,200 professionals hold dual certification. Because speech-language pathologists and audiologists are autonomous professionals, people can

DEPARTMENT OF LABOR DEFINITIONS

The Department of Labor has defined the profession of speech-language pathology and audiology as follows:

076.101–010   Audiologist (profess. & kin.)

Specializes in diagnostic evaluation of hearing, prevention, habilitative and rehabilitative services for auditory problems, and research related to hearing and attendant disorders: Determines range, nature, and degree of hearing function related to patient's auditory efficiency (communication needs), using electro-acoustic instrumentation, such as pure-tone and speech audiometers, and acoustic impedance equipment. Coordinates audiometric results with other diagnostic data, such as educational, medical, social, and behavioral information. Differentiates between organic and nonorganic hearing disabilities through evaluation of total response pattern and use of acoustic tests, such as Stenger and electrodermal audiometry. Plans, directs, conducts, or participates in conservation, habilitative and rehabilitative programs including hearing aid selection and orientation, counseling, guidance, auditory training, speech reading, language habilitation, and speech conservation. May conduct research in physiology, pathology, biophysics, and psychophysics of auditory systems. May design and develop clinical and research procedures and apparatus. May act as consultant to educational, medical, and other professional groups. May teach art and

science of audiology and direct scientific projects. May specialize in fields, such as industrial audiology, geriatric audiology, pediatric audiology, and research audiology.

076.107–010   Speech Pathologists (profess. & kin.) speech clinician; speech therapist

Specializes in diagnosis and treatment of speech and language problems, and engages in scientific study of human communication: Diagnoses and evaluates speech and language competencies of individuals, including assessment of speech and language skills as related to educational, medical, social, and psychological factors. Plans, directs, or conducts habilitative and rehabilitative treatment programs to restore communicative efficiency of individuals with communication problems of organic and nonorganic etiology. Provides counseling and guidance to speech and language handicapped individuals. May act as consultant to educational, medical, and other professional groups. May teach scientific principles of human communication. May direct scientific projects investigating biophysical and biosocial phenomena associated with voice, speech, and language. May conduct research to develop diagnostic and remedial techniques or design apparatus.

FROM: *Dictionary of Occupational Titles 1977,* Fourth Edition, U.S. Department of Labor.

obtain their services directly rather than having to be referred by a physician. More information about licensure is in the June 1986 "State Licensure" issue of *Asha*. The report of the Ad Hoc Committee on Professional Autonomy was published in the May 1986 issue of *Asha*.

Clinical practice today requires that all clinicians know at least basic information about licensure and scope-of-practice issues, professional liability, business, and contracts. As we have become an autonomous and a largely licensed and/or certified group of practitioners, we have also gained more legal responsibilities. Ten years ago, few speech-language pathologists would have been interested in reading about liability and liability insurance. We often associated malpractice and liability issues with physicians. There has been a lot of publicity about skyrocketing malpractice insurance costs and the increasing number of claims filed against all types of medical specialists, especially obstetricians. However, in today's litigious society, all health professionals are—or should be—interested in protecting themselves against potential lawsuits. Our increasing involvement in working with individuals who have dysphagia, and in "hands-on" procedures for laryngectomee rehabilitation increase the necessity for liability insurance. ASHA offers a liability insurance policy through Albert H. Wohlers Company. (For more information, write or call Albert H. Wohlers Company, 1500 Higgins Road, Park Ridge, IL 60068; phone [800] 323–2106.)

We hope that you will never experience a lawsuit or complaint against your professional practice and behavior. Adherence to the scope of practice established by your state's licensure law and to ASHA's Code of Ethics is a good way to avoid problems. You can further protect yourself by obtaining liability insurance, maintaining currency in the field, and monitoring standards and liability trends. There are, however, no guarantees. Liability is a hazard of professional practice in all health fields and will continue to receive a great deal of attention. For more information, refer to Miller and Lubinski (1986); Lynch (1986); and Silverman (1983).

In 1983 the American Speech-Language Hearing Association adopted the following terminology and definitions regarding the knowledge base that underlies professional practice and the forms of professional practice that evolve from the discipline:

ASHA TERMINOLOGY AND DEFINITIONS

The Discipline: The branch of knowledge, both theoretical and applied, that deals with human communication sciences and disorders. The discipline shall be called human communication sciences and disorders.

The Profession: The application of the discipline in professional endeavors which are based fundamentally on the study of the discipline. These professional endeavors may take three major forms:

ASHA TERMINOLOGY AND DEFINITIONS *Continued*

1. clinical services for individuals with speech-language-hearing disorders, aimed at the amelioration of communication difficulties stemming from such disorders;

2. research aimed at expanding knowledge about human communication, human communication disorders, and/or effective amelioration strategies; and

3. teaching/supervising persons in human communication sciences and disorders.

The Core of Knowledge: The domain of study integral to the profession, where all aspects of human communication and its disorders are viewed as interdependent; the knowledge common to all members of the profession.

Designated Areas of Practice: The identifiable ranges of clinical services for individuals with speech-language-hearing disorders; applies particularly (but not necessarily exclusively) to entry-level competencies. Although each designated area of practice identifies a primary focus of clinical endeavor, areas may overlap and intersect. Currently, two designated areas of clinical practice are (1) speech-language pathology, and (2) audiology.

Specialty: Expertise within the scope of a designated area of practice; refers to competencies beyond those expected at entry-level, pursued at the option of the individual. (ASHA Executive Board)

Recognizing that speech-language pathology and audiology are the same profession, we have chosen to focus the remainder of this book on the area of practice of speech-language pathology (SLP). This decision does not intend to place audiology in a lesser role; rather, we believe that each area of practice is worthy of its own book. Certain chapters of this work will be applicable to both speech-language pathology and audiology, but our mission is to provide a comprehensive introduction to the clinical practice of speech-language pathology. Some of the activities, concerns, trends, and issues related to audiology are discussed in articles cited at the end of this chapter. A short description of audiology services is also provided in Appendix A.

PROFESSIONAL ASSOCIATIONS, PROGRAMS, POLICIES, AND PUBLICATIONS

American Speech-Language-Hearing Association

Mission and Membership

The American Speech-Language-Hearing Association, founded in 1925, is a scholarly and professional organization. Its 50,000 members are speech-language pathologists and/or audiologists who have earned a master's degree or its equivalent in speech-language pathology; audiology; or speech, language, and hearing science and hold the Certificate of Clinical Competence. Some members hold graduate degrees in other fields but conduct research or pursue other special interests in the field of human communication. Members who provide clinical services must hold the Certificate of Clinical Competence in either speech-language pathology (CCC-SLP) or audiology (CCC-A).

It is also possible to hold a Certificate of Clinical Competence without membership in ASHA, but an individual then has none of the rights and privileges of membership. Certificate holders pay a one-time application fee as well as an annual fee to maintain certification status. Members of ASHA pay initial membership and certification fees as well as annual dues. The amount of fees and dues is established by the Legislative Council.

According to ASHA Bylaws (1986), the purposes of the association are to

> Encourage basic scientific study of the processes of individual human communication, with special reference to speech, hearing and language, promote investigation and prevention of disorders of human communication, and foster improvement of clinical procedures with such disorders; to stimulate exchange of information among persons and organizations thus engaged, and to disseminate such information.

Standards

In addition to its individual certification program, administered by the Clinical Certification Board (CCB), ASHA also conducts standards programs for education and training institutions and clinical service facilities. The Professional Services Board (PSB) reviews and accredits service delivery programs; the Educational Standards Board (ESB) accredits educational programs. ESB is recognized by the Council on Postsecondary Education (COPA) as the sole accrediting body for speech-language pathology and audiology educational programs. It is also recognized by the U.S. Department of Education. More information about ASHA's standards programs is found in chapter 8.

Organization and Management

ASHA is managed by the Executive Board, which implements policies established by the Legislative Council and stated in the Bylaws. The Executive Board is composed of the president of ASHA (who serves a one-year term), and president-elect, past president, all the vice-presidents, and the executive director. The executive director of the association is the only salaried member of the Executive Board and does not vote. Each vice-president represents one of six areas: administration, clinical affairs, education and scientific affairs, planning, professional and governmental affairs, and standards and ethics.

The Legislative Council governs the association. Councilors are nominated and elected by members from each of the states and from among those members who live outside the United States. The Council meets during ASHA annual conventions and may also hold additional gatherings. The Committee on Resolutions initiates resolutions, considers submissions from the membership, and classifies resolutions according to topic areas for which Coordinating Committee chairs are responsible. As representatives of the ASHA membership, councilors debate and vote on resolutions. Approved resolutions become official policies or procedures of the association.

Members of ASHA have the opportunity to serve on a number of standing or ad hoc committees and boards. Most of these committees report to ASHA vice-presidents according to responsibility area: administration, clinical affairs, education and scientific affairs, planning, professional and governmental affairs, and standards and ethics. Committees on credentials, honors, nominations, resolutions, special rules, and the Legislative Council Handbook report directly to the Legislative Council. Members who wish to be considered for appointments submit a Committee Pool Data Form (published annually in *Asha*) to the Committee on Committees, which reports to the Executive Board. A complete list of all ASHA committees and boards is also published annually in *Asha*. Because there are far more applications than positions in any given year, members may have to resubmit requests for several years or more.

Additional opportunities to serve the association include the Congressional Action Contact Network, the Insurance Consultant Network, and the Minority Concerns Collective. There are also Related Professional Organizations (RPOs), such as the Public School Caucus and the Council of University Supervisors in Speech-Language Pathology and Audiology (CUSPSPA), a network of university supervisors whose interests pertain to a specific employment setting or responsibility area. Information about any of these groups may be obtained by contacting the ASHA National Office.

The National Office

ASHA's headquarters, or the ASHA National Office, is located at 10801 Rockville Pike, Rockville, Maryland 20852 (a suburb of Washington, D.C.). Its telephone number is (301) 897–5700. The ASHA Actionline number is (800) 638–6868. Members may call the toll-free Actionline to inquire about a variety of issues (e.g., journals, certification and dues information, or referral to appropriate staff members).

The work of more than 140 staff members is supervised by the Executive Director, who is assisted by directors of administration, business management, governmental affairs, professional affairs, and public information departments. National office staff coordinate the activities of the association and implement policies and programs as designated by the Legislative Council and the Executive Board. Activities of the staff are published annually in *Asha* and in the annual report of the association.

Honors

ASHA members who have distinguished themselves through professional or scientific achievement may be nominated for Fellowship by another ASHA member (sponsor), seconded by two ASHA Fellows designated as cosponsors. The Committee on Honors approves nominees for Fellowship by a two-thirds vote. Criteria for election include outstanding contributions to the profession in at least three areas from among clinical services, academic teaching, research and publications, administration, service to ASHA, state and local speech-language-hearing association activities, or efforts for related organizations.

Individuals who have made outstanding contributions to ASHA may be awarded the Honors of the Association upon recommendation of the Committee on Honors and a three-fourths vote of the Legislative Council. This award is the highest bestowed by our professional organization.

ASHA's Continuing Education Program

In 1979, ASHA initiated a voluntary program of continuing education after more than a decade of study, debate, and revision of Executive Board and Legislative Council resolutions. The program was introduced in two phases: Phase I included development of a system for approving continuing education sponsors and the development of the Award for Continuing Education (ACE); Phase II, ratified by the Legislative Council in 1982, expanded the association's continuing education program to include development of a wider variety of approved activities (e.g., self-study, telecourses).

ASHA maintains a registry of each participant's continuing education activities. Each time a participant completes an activity he or she pays a fee, and a computer form is sent to the registry service. A cumulative record is available to participants to track their own activities as well as to document participation for those who wish to earn the Award for Continuing Education (ACE). Requirements for the ACE may be revised periodically. Currently, an ACE can be earned by meeting one of several types of requirements: (1) accrue seven continuing education units (CEUs) from approved sponsors (ASHA's Continuing Education Section maintains a list of approved sponsors); (2) complete six semester hours (nine quarter hours) of academic coursework from an approved sponsor or graduate program accredited by the Educational Standards Board (ESB); (3) earn a combination of CEUs and academic credit; (4) retake the National Examination in Speech-Language Pathology and/or Audiology not sooner than three years after the previous examination was passed. There are specific requirements for the content of academic coursework, encompassing basic communication processes and various professional areas. Certain ratios apply to the combination CEU–academic coursework option. Complete details, instructions, and application forms can be obtained by calling or writing the Continuing Education Section at the ASHA National Office. ACE requirements and other information related to continuing education activities are also published periodically in the journal *Asha*.

During its meeting at the 1986 ASHA annual convention, the Legislative Council supported in principle the development of a plan for specialty recognition. This plan is to be based upon the establishment of sections focused on major areas of clinical and research interest (e.g., language acquisition and disorders of language acquisition, voice and voice disorders, speech physiology and disorders, rehabilitation of the hearing impaired, cultural linguistic diversity, administration, professional education and supervision, and many others). It will provide for the eventual implementation of affiliation in particular sections for interested ASHA members, a mechanism for recognition of expertise within the interest area encompassed by each section, and opportunities to identify areas of more specialized interest within the broader dimensions described by section participants. The plan is to be further developed and presented to the 1987 Legislative Council for approval.

Although ASHA's program of continuing education is voluntary, 15 of the 36 states that have enacted licensing laws for speech-language pathologists and audiologists require continuing education for license renewal. There is a wide variation in the number and type of required hours or units (10 hours equal one continuing education unit, or CEU). For example, Florida requires one CEU in one year, whereas Georgia requires 40 hours or four CEUs in two years. North Dakota requires six clock hours in one year. ASHA CEUs are accepted by all states that require continuing education to maintain licensure. Continuing education requirements may change, so it is important to keep informed of all requirements related to licensure in your state.

Publications

All ASHA members receive four journals. Articles of broad professional interest in speech-language pathology or audiology are published monthly in *Asha*, which also serves as the official voice of the association.

The *Journal of Speech and Hearing Disorders (JSHD)* is published four times a year. It addresses the nature and treatment of speech, hearing, and language disorders and the clinical and supervisory processes involved in assessment and treatment.

The *Journal of Speech and Hearing Research (JSHR)*, also produced quarterly, publishes reports of experimental studies pertaining to normal processes and disorders of speech, hearing, and language.

Language, Speech and Hearing Services in Schools (LSHSS) focuses on information about speech, language, and hearing services for children, particularly in school settings.

The *Governmental Affairs Review (GAR)*, published quarterly by ASHA's Governmental Affairs Department, is not included in membership benefits but may be ordered for a reasonable annual fee. This periodical covers recent federal legislation, actions of regulatory agencies, reimbursement policies, and judicial decisions affecting communicatively impaired persons, speech-language pathologists, and audiologists.

ASHA also produces many other publications that may be ordered by mail or telephone. Some of the items available include monographs, film catalogs, teleconference tapes, special reports, manuals, directories, indexes, guides, pamphlets, and brochures. Information about publications is sent regularly to the ASHA membership. Interested persons should direct inquiries to the office of Publication Sales at the ASHA National Office address.

Other periodicals of interest to speech-language pathologists and audiologists are listed in Appendix B. This appendix also contains a list of many associations, foundations, and organizations related to the concerns and activities of the speech-language pathology and audiology profession.

American Speech-Language-Hearing Foundation (ASHF)

Established in 1956, ASHF is a charitable trust designed to advance scientific and educational endeavor in speech-language pathology and audiology. The only foundation dedicated to all communicatively impaired persons, ASHF focuses on the professionals who serve these individuals. Activities include support of research efforts of students, new PhDs, and senior investigators; awards for clinical achievement; scholarships; and sponsorship of an annual computer conference and financial planning seminars for ASHA members. Information about ASHF may be obtained by contacting the ASHA National Office.

National Association for Hearing and Speech Action (NASHA)

NASHA is the consumer affiliate of the American Speech-Language-Hearing Association. It is a consumer information, action, and referral service and publishes consumer-oriented information. The number for NASHA's helpline for consumers is (803) 638–6255. The business telephone number is (301) 897–8682.

National Student Speech-Language-Hearing Association (NSSLHA)

NSSLHA is the student affiliate of ASHA. This organization has an elected executive council and annual dues, and publishes the *Nsslha Journal* once a year, as well as topical monographs. The Executive Council consists of 15 members, 10 regional councilors who are students representing local chapters, and five consultants (ASHA members). There is also an administrative consultant. Officers are elected from among the student councilors. Most speech-language pathology and audiology training programs have local chapters of NSSLHA. Advisors are usually faculty members.

An important benefit of NSSLHA membership is the reduction offered for initial ASHA membership and certification fees. Additionally, NSSLHA members receive all the professional journals sent to ASHA members.

International Association of Logopedics and Phoniatrics (IALP)

Founded in 1924, the IALP's purpose is to promote the scientific study of disorders of human communication. There are 50 affiliated societies (including ASHA) in 34 countries. IALP holds a triennial convention and publishes a bimonthly journal, *Folia Phoniatricia*. The address of the International Association of Logopedics and Phoniatrics is Avenue de la Gare 6, CH–1003 Lausanne, Switzerland.

State Speech-Language-Hearing Associations

Many speech-language pathologists and audiologists are members of state speech-language-hearing associations. These groups have elected officers, standing and ad hoc committees, and annual membership dues. They sponsor annual meetings, conferences, and continuing education opportunities. Additionally, members advocate legislative and regulatory changes (e.g., Medicaid, licensure, state education agency policies, education issues) that will create and/or maintain favorable conditions for professional practice in individual states and localities.

Many state associations publish journals, newsletters, and other materials; some groups hire executive staff. The Council of State Association Presidents (CSAP) is an organization of officers of state speech-language-hearing associations. Its purpose is to collect and coordinate information exchanged between state associations and to promote communication on professional matters between state associations and ASHA as well as related professional organizations.

ACTIVITIES

1. Ask faculty, staff, and/or fellow students to identify the professional title (e.g., speech clinician, speech pathologist) they prefer and/or use.

2. Compare results obtained in activity 1 with responses to a second survey conducted with any or all of the following groups:
   a. physicians
   b. clients or parents of clients
   c. teachers
   d. psychologists
   e. allied health professionals (physical therapists, occupational therapists, nurses, social workers)

3. Contact a local, state, and/or national speech and hearing association and inquire about the benefits of becoming a member.

4. Review an ASHA membership application. Discuss with your academic instructor or with the coordinator of clinic practice the schedule you will follow during your graduate program in order to satisfy requirements for ASHA membership.

5. Identify at least two clinical populations or content areas you may wish to concentrate on during your graduate program. Select two periodicals from Appendix B that address issues relevant to your particular interests. Read one article in each of the most current issues of these journals.

6. Review the convention speeches of the last five ASHA presidents. These should provide a perspective on current and future issues facing the profession of speech-language pathology and audiology.

7. Pursue information about the NSSLHA chapter on your campus. Consider joining this group or establishing a local chapter if one is not presently active.

8. Identify the current presidents of ASHA, NSSLHA, and your state organization.

9. Determine when your state convention will be held and mark your calendar. Perhaps you could volunteer to help with the planning of the meeting.

10. Think of someone in the profession you would like to hear speak at your state convention. Contact the association's program chairperson and offer your suggestion.

REFERENCES

ASHA Ad Hoc Committee on Professional Autonomy. (1986). The autonomy of speech-language pathology and audiology. *Asha, 28*(5), 53–57.

Hyman, C. (1987). *Demographic Profile of the ASHA Membership.* Rockville, MD: ASHA Research Division/Demographic Branch.

Lynch, C. (1986). Harm to the public: Is it real? *Asha, 28*(6), 25–31.

Malone, R. (1986). Comment section. *Asha, 28*(5), 2.

Miller, T., & Lubinski, R. (1986). Professional liability in speech-language pathology and audiology. *Asha, 28*(6), 45–47.

Sarnecky, E. (1987, February 18). Speech-language pathology and audiology: A profession that lets you be what you want to be. *Career and Higher Education News, 1* (3).

Silverman, F. (1983). *Legal aspects of speech-language pathology: An overview of law for clinicians, researchers, and teachers.* Englewood Cliffs, NJ: Prentice-Hall.

Taylor, J. S. (1981). *Speech-language pathology services in the schools.* New York: Grune & Stratton.

CHAPTER TWO

Clinical Practice Settings

INTRODUCTION

Those of us who attended graduate school in the early seventies had very definite ideas about the life-style of a speech-language pathologist. Our images or illusions were based, in part, on the promise of vast and varied employment settings, and all seemed idyllic—the glamour of working in a hospital, the stimulation of an academic career, the charm and flexibility of serving school children. With these images firmly in mind we have worked in the public schools, hospitals, universities, clinics, businesses, and the ASHA National Office. We have taught, facilitated, consulted, researched, supervised, written, retrained, directed, and collaborated. If the monetary gains were small, the intellectual and experiential rewards were great. Over the years we have maintained our enthusiasm for and commitment to the field but have also developed a better, perhaps more mature (or at least middle-aged), view of the pleasures and discomforts derived from our work.

We are reluctant to provide a profile of the "typical" speech-language pathologist, but demographic data of the ASHA membership suggest that the majority of practitioners hold master's degrees and the Certificate of Clinical Competence in Speech-Language Pathology, are licensed by the state in which they practice, are engaged in clinical service, work full-time for an educational institution, and are white females in their early thirties.

The preceding description by no means characterizes a great many speech-language-hearing professionals, who work in virtually all health and educational settings. Some employment locations include hospitals, rehabilitation centers, skilled nursing facilities, hospices, government agencies, community clinics, universities, private offices, and home health agencies.

Salaries for speech-language-hearing professionals vary by certification status, employment setting and primary activity, highest academic degree held, geographic region, and length of professional experience. ASHA members who are engaged in administration, college teaching, and research activities earn the highest median annual salaries; those who work in schools, the lowest. In between, in descending order, are personnel in government agencies, private practices, and nongovernment health settings. Members who have doctoral degrees earn 64% more than those who hold master's degrees (based on median salary). Professionals who are dually certified earn higher salaries on the average than single-certificate holders (CCC-SLP or CCC-A). Audiologists have higher mean salaries than speech-language pathologists (Hyman, 1986).

As the general population ages and more rehabilitation services are needed, the outlook for employment in the speech-language-hearing profession is very good. In fact, it is anticipated that professional services including optometry, podiatry, chiropractic, private-duty nursing, occupational and physical therapy, and speech-language pathology and audiology will grow at a faster rate than most other personal health services ("Education of the Handicapped Act becomes law," 1986). The future is not without its challenges, however, as the health-care system becomes increasingly controlled by purchasers and payers, (i.e., employers and insurance companies), as other health professionals offer services to communicatively impaired persons, and as government funding continues to decrease. These issues as well as a number of others facing the profession are discussed at length in succeeding chapters.

In the remainder of this discussion on employment we will share our knowledge and experience and a touch of our dreams in describing employment opportunities in speech-language pathology. We discuss the most common work settings for speech-language pathologists: schools, universities, private practice, and health care (hospitals, nursing homes, home health services, community clinics, and health maintenance organizations).

EMPLOYMENT SETTINGS

Schools

The school speech-language pathologist is one of the most visible members of the profession. Recent legislative reforms have literally placed the school clinician on the front line in providing speech, language, and hearing services to children and in acting as a catalyst to improve existing programs and initiate new ones.

In the United States clinical services began in the public schools under the title of speech improvement or speech correction programs. Today, more than 40% of the ASHA membership is employed in a school setting (Hyman, 1986). Yet, in reference to school clinicians, Maxwell (1986) comments that "the nature of their specialized roles and contributions to the field is frequently unclear and in some settings remains unacknowledged" (p. 26).

The stereotype of a school speech-language pathologist is one of an itinerant clinician whose primary task is to provide group therapy to children with functional articulation problems. This view is neither current nor complete. According to a 1984 ASHA Omnibus Survey, 52.2% of the caseload was identified as having a primary disorder of language as compared to 34.8% described as articulation disordered. This is in sharp contrast to a 1960 survey that identified 81% of those serviced in the schools as articulation disordered and 4.5% as language impaired (Eger, 1986). Table 2.1 contains data on trends in national and local caseloads for six categories of speech and language disorders over the past 35 years (Eger, 1986). Although the numbers of articulation-disordered children remain relatively high, they have been decreasing steadily. Further, the proportion of direct therapy time allotted articulation-impaired children has been adjusted to accommodate a more diverse population and to include the more severely and profoundly handicapped, the bilingual, the dialectally different, the preschool population, and the junior high and high school students, all who may present a broad spectrum of speech, language, voice, and fluency problems. Two significant factors in this shift in caseload emphasis were the increased recognition of and regard for language learning disabled children and the implementation of PL 94–142 (Sommers & Hatton, 1985). These factors contributed to so many important changes in session frequency and duration and in the creation of new and/or alternative service delivery options that Sommers and Hatton suggest we may be witnessing an "evolution in scheduling" (1985, p. 291).

The passage in 1975 of PL 94–142, the Education for All Handicapped Children Act, carried with it the mandate that each local school system create a plan for the provision of an appropriate public education to handicapped children, including the communicatively handicapped. The implications of this legislation for the speech-language pathologist working in the schools have been significant. Previously serviced through health and medical facilities, many handicapped children, including the severely impaired and the multiply handicapped, are now "mainstreamed," or provided an education and special assistance in regular schools. The requirement that children be educated in the least-restrictive environment has expanded the population served by school speech-language pathologists, led to the elaboration of program alternatives, and influenced service delivery models.

In January 1981 the ASHA Committee on Language, Speech, and Hearing Services in the Schools drafted guidelines on mandated caseload requirements in the schools, as membership surveys consistently pointed to caseload selection and size as the primary concerns of speech-language pathologists employed in school settings. Thirty states specified a maximum caseload ranging from 20 to

TABLE 2.1

Caseload Breakdown (%) Nationally (ASHA) and Locally (AIU)

Disorder Type	1960 (Schools, N = 1462)[a] ASHA	1981 (N = 899)[b] ASHA	1982 Omnibus (Schools, N = 295)[c] ASHA	1984 Omnibus (Schools, N = 565)[d] ASHA	1984 ISHA (N = 1103)[e]	1984–85 School Year Allegheny IU (N = 93)	1985–86 School Year Allegheny IU (N = 93)
Articulation	81.0%	47.0%	33.0%	34.8%	37.0%	45.5%	41.5%
Language	4.5%	46.7%	52.4%	52.2%	55.0%	45.4%*	49.8%*
Fluency	6.5%	3.9%	4.3%	4.1%	3.0%	2.8%	2.9%
Voice	2.3%	2.3%	2.5%	2.4%	1.5%	1.0%	1.0%
Hearing	2.5%	0	5.4%	4.5%	0	3.5%	3.0%
Other	3.2%	0	2.5%	2.0%	4.5%	1.8%	1.8%

a. Public School Speech and Hearing Services, ASHA Monograph Supplement No. 8, 1961.
b. Survey of Services in the Public Schools, Government Affairs Review, Fall 1981.
c. Fein, D. J. (1983). Survey Report: 1982 Omnibus, Asha, 25(3), 53–57.
d. ASHA 1984 Omnibus Survey.
e. Block, F. K., Illinois Speech-Language-Hearing Association School Survey, 1984.

*Includes students who have both language and articulation problems.

NOTE: From School Issues: Gaining Support for Your Program [ASHA Teleconference] by D. L. Eger, October 10, 1986, Rockville, MD: ASHA. Copyright 1986 by ASHA. Reprinted by permission.

110, with an average caseload of 43 during the week the survey was completed (Eger, 1986). The committee also recommended four models for service delivery in the schools: indirect-service/consultation, direct-service/itinerant, direct-service/resource-room, and direct-service/self-contained. Brief descriptions of these service options are provided in the accompanying box. The committee report of 1983 and articles by Frassinelli, Superior, and Meyers, (1983) and Pickering (1981) contain more complete definitions and interpretations of these treatment models.

The size, needs, and structure of the local school district often determine the organizational model used. The majority of speech-language pathologists employed in the schools work on an itinerant basis (Digest of Education Statistics, 1983–84). The itinerant model involves traveling to different buildings and scheduling children a certain number of sessions per week over a period of time. Some speech-language pathologists are assigned to a single school. School clinicians also work in special classes, resource rooms, or self-contained classrooms. Others may be either full- or part-time members of the pupil-evaluation team. Speech-language pathologists may function as resource consultants to teachers, administrators, and other school staff. Finally, some may be employed as supervisors or administrators of speech and language programs.

The publication *Project Upgrade: Model Regulations for School Language, Speech, and Hearing Programs and Services* (Jones & Healey, 1973) offers recommendations for service delivery options. Its authors discourage the sole use of the itinerant model or any other single method for delivery of service to the school population with communication disorders. The types of service options or school-placement alternatives offered are diagnostic centers, full-time special classes, regular classroom placement with supportive or related services, direct or indirect services to pupils provided through resource rooms, consultative services to regular or special classroom teachers, home-bound and/or hospitals services, parent-infant instruction services, and residential programs. For complete descriptions of these services refer to Jones and Healey (1973), Neidecker (1980), or Flowers, (1984).

With the recent adoption of PL 99–457, which is an amendment to the Education for All Handicapped Children Act, school programs will probably continue to expand, diversify, and flourish. This law requires appropriate early intervention services to all handicapped infants, toddlers, and their families. Although the full impact of this legislation has yet to be realized, PL 99–457 will undoubtedly strengthen the position of public schools as providers of comprehensive services to handicapped infants and young children and may make the term *preschooler* somewhat of a misnomer.

Changes in caseload composition and numbers have also resulted in changes in the qualifications required of the service providers themselves, that is, the school speech-language pathologists and audiologists. Although some speech-language pathologists in the schools are working at a bachelor's degree level, the increased specialization and skills necessary to serve today's school population have led many to conclude that a master's degree should be mandatory. In fact, a new part *H* of PL 94–142 will require those states that now have lower standards

SERVICE DELIVERY MODELS IN PUBLIC SCHOOL SPEECH-LANGUAGE PATHOLOGY PROGRAMS

Indirect-Service Consultation Model

The *consultation* model is indirect because the speech-language pathologist trains someone else (other professionals, classroom teachers, or parents) to carry out the program established and evaluated by the speech-language pathologist. Frassinelli, Superior, and Meyers (1983) described this model as "a three person chain of service in which a consultant interacts with a caregiver to benefit an individual for whom the caregiver is responsible" (p. 25).

Pickering (1981) outlined a consultation model for school speech-language pathologist and classroom-teacher collaboration. This model offered not only objectives for both the child and the teacher to improve communication skills, but also suggestions for the consultant as an instructor, a specialist, and a facilitator.

Direct-Service/Itinerant Model

The *itinerant* model serves students who are usually placed in regular or special classrooms but are seen for speech or language therapy outside that environment, either for individual or small-group sessions. Larger caseloads are often served with this model. A variation of this model may include speech-language pathology services within the classroom involving some elements of teacher consultation/ collaboration.

Direct-Service/Resource-Room Model

In the *resource-room* model, the stu-

dent's academic objectives are often included in speech-language goals and activities. Designed for students who present more severe communication disorders, this model may be used to help the individual work on self-instructional materials and to structure individual or small-group sessions with the speech-language pathologist. For this model the committee recommended a maximum caseload of 15 to 25 persons.

Direct-Service/Self-Contained Model

The *self-contained* model has been designed primarily for children with severe language disorders, but it may also be used for groups of children who present other severe communication disorders that require special all-day class placement. In addition to planning, implementing, and evaluating communication goals, the speech-language pathologist also serves as the classroom teacher in this model. For inclusion in this program, the child must be assessed as having *primary* educational and/or social needs in the area of communication (for example, a diagnosis as being emotionally, mentally, or hearing impaired). The maximum recommended caseload is up to 10 children without a classroom aide and 15 with an aide.

NOTE: Descriptions were based on the recommendations of the Committee on Language, Speech, and Hearing Services in the Schools (ASHA, 1983).

(BA level) for school personnel (Alabama, Arkansas, Florida, Georgia, Louisiana, Maine, Maryland, Nevada, New Jersey, New York, North Dakota, Oklahoma, Oregon, Pennsylvania, Rhode Island, South Carolina, Tennessee, Utah, Virginia, and Wyoming) to raise the educational standards of school personnel to levels commensurate with professionals servicing nonschool populations. This means that the MA degree will become the standard for speech-language pathologists and audiologists employed in schools, except in Alaska, Arizona, the District of Columbia, Minnesota, and South Dakota, where neither licensure nor MA certification is required ("Education of the Handicapped Act becomes law," 1986).

In addition to a master's degree, speech-language pathologists who work in schools should also be required to hold both a license in the state where they practice (if applicable) and a teaching certificate. Requirements for the Certificate of Clinical Competence issued by the American Speech-Language-Hearing Association usually accompany licensure standards.

Despite the variety of opportunities available in the schools, some individuals are apprehensive about employment in this setting. In fact, several of the issues and concerns of the 1960s—large caseloads in some states, lack of materials in some districts, inadequate or inappropriate workspaces, bureaucratic requirements, the need to travel from school to school, the requisites of teacher certification and membership in a teacher union—still are problems for a number of speech-language pathologists in the 1980s. Unfortunately, continued differences—whether real or imagined—in school clinicians' educational levels and in levels needed to cope with the severity of the problems among the populations they serve have contributed to a low-prestige professional image. In addition, the implementation of certain educational reforms, specifically PL 94–142, has increased the amount of paperwork required by school administrators; and some clinicians view the requirements as excessive and burdensome.

These drawbacks must be weighed against the advantages of a good benefits program, relatively long vacations, comparatively short workdays, opportunities for advancement in some larger school systems and service centers, and opportunities for continuing education and staff development. Further, the qualifications and responsibilities of speech-language pathologists in the schools have changed markedly. In addition, the energy, commitment, enthusiasm, and creativity of public school practitioners have earned a superior reputation for many speech-language-hearing programs in schools across the country. According to *Asha* staff members, "A sample of those programs and services in public schools, the new, the more traditional, those backed by the resources of a school district, and those run on individual inspiration, shows speech-language-hearing services in the public schools taking new approaches to continuing problems and improving on existing programs" (Staff, 1986, p. 18). Trends toward integration of speech-language services with classroom programs, naturalistic assessment and intervention, inclusion of parents and peers in therapy and generalization activities, interdisciplinary and transdisciplinary assessment, early intervention and prevention, and use of communication assistants are becoming realities.

Sally Maxwell, chairperson of the Public School Caucus, a support group and information network that promotes and assists members' efforts to heighten local and national attention on relevant school issues, asserts that "nowhere else can a professional have such a 'holistic' impact upon the development of children as they learn how to communicate effectively within society" (1986, p. 26). It would appear that school speech-language pathologists, who have historically been the mainstay of our profession, may move to the forefront in providing services to communication-handicapped children of all ages.

Colleges and Universities

Individuals who are attracted to a faculty career are likely to have a strong interest in research and/or clinical or classroom teaching but wish to maintain an identity close to the discipline of speech-language pathology or audiology. Incentives such as sabbatical and leave policies, number of vacations and holidays, flexible schedules, possibility of part-time employment, opportunities for professional involvement and development, opportunities for consultation with compensation and extra paid teaching assignments may also serve to attract and retain productive faculty. As Wilson suggested in 1942, the primary reward of a university appointment, compared with other professions requiring equal training, is prestige. This may still be true today.

It is important to examine not only the benefits of a faculty appointment but some of the problems as well. Universities have traditionally confronted a number of thorny issues, which have perhaps added to the charm if not the challenge of this setting. Ideally, faculty members might have the chance to combine their talents and interests in teaching, research and supervision, or administration. Persons entering the academic profession quickly discover, however, that "disciplinary tasks" such as conducting research, developing grant proposals, and training of future researchers, and "institutional duties" of teaching, advising, supervising, and participating in administration are not equally valued (Light, Mardsen, & Corl, 1973). In the current milieu, recognition and promotion go to those who are most successful in obtaining grants and publishing research and may not correlate with teaching ability or clinical competence.

The traditional academic career follows the progression of instructor, assistant professor, associate professor, and professor. Tenure is a status granted faculty members who demonstrate scholarship and achievement in such areas as research and teaching in their field. In the case of an individual whose speciality is speech-language pathology, there are additional clinical and administrative opportunities such as supervision of clinical practice, coordination of clinical education, and direction of university training clinics. Through the efforts of groups such as the Council of University Supervisors of Practicum in Speech-Language Pathology and Audiology (CUSPSPA), clinical supervision is becoming recognized as a legitimate area of expertise and practice. Increased attention has been focused on the academic preparation, clinical skills, and professional experience necessary for supervisory personnel. The ASHA Committee on Supervision has led an active campaign to establish minimal qualifications for clinical supervisors (1982, 1985).

Individuals who aspire to a faculty career in speech-language pathology begin with a bachelor's degree and then complete graduate school. For some, the master's degree is sufficient for obtaining a teaching or supervisory appointment. However, at many colleges and most universities a master's level individual faces limited opportunity for advancement unless promoted in title (e.g., clinical supervisor is advanced to assistant clinic director, and then clinic director) rather than in academic rank. The standard faculty career clearly favors those who hold a doctoral degree.

In the 1985–86 academic year there were 293 graduate programs in speech-language pathology and/or audiology. Many of these programs sponsor their own training centers. In fact, college and university clinics represent the second oldest type of American service delivery programs in our field. The principle goals of most of these clinics are (1) to offer clinical instruction to students in speech-language pathology and audiology, (2) to provide clinical services for persons with communication problems, and (3) to continue investigation of the nature and management of communication problems. To enable students to fulfill their clinical practicum requirements, most of the clinical services are provided by students who work under the direct supervision of faculty or staff supervisors. "The major responsibility of the clinical staff in a training program is to provide sensitive supervision of student clinicians in an environment supportive to the professional development of each individual; and, at the same time, to provide an exemplary model to motivate the student toward clinical excellence" (Hardick & Oyer, 1987).

The population seeking and receiving services at university clinics is likely to include individuals who present a wide variety of speech, language, and hearing problems. Faculty who have established reputations as specialists with particular disorder groups may attract individuals with these problems from a broad geographic area to a particular campus. University-subsidized clinics may also be in a unique position to serve the indigent, long-term cases such as the mentally retarded or developmentally disabled and those with progressive illnesses such as Alzheimer's or Parkinson's disease. Given the amount and diversity of expertise represented on a university faculty, there is frequent opportunity for consultation, demonstration therapy, family counseling, and clinical research.

Because university clinics are outpatient facilities, however, clients are least likely to be in need of services associated with problems of an acute, medical nature (e.g., early stages of aphasia). After discharge, these persons may prefer to continue with their treatment at the hospitals where they first received medical care. Alternatively, they may be placed in rehabilitation centers, chronic-care facilities, or, if more appropriate, receive help through home health agencies. Hardick and Oyer (1987) suggest that the primary differences between university-based speech and hearing clinics and other programs are related to the former's primary mission of professional education of speech-language pathologists and audiologists. Other distinctions noted include departmental and fiscal organization, personnel structure, financial management, and client scheduling (Flower, 1984; Hardick & Oyer, 1987).

Departments of communication disorders may be located in colleges of education, arts and sciences, allied health professions, or medicine, exemplifying the various interpretations and/or wide scope of the discipline as viewed by its own members and by institutional administrators and trustees. Although programs may be influenced by the schools in which they are housed, some degree of similarity is to be expected as a by-product of accreditation standards and licensure and certification requirements.

According to Hyman (1987), a relatively small proportion of speech-language pathologists and audiologists engage in research and teaching as their primary employment activities. The limited number of ASHA members primarily employed in colleges or university teaching (4.4%) or research (1.3%) may be based in part on the relative scarcity of individuals holding doctoral degrees as well as the relatively small number of speech-language pathology and audiology departments in colleges and universities. Despite the disproportionately low representation of college- and university-employed speech-language pathologists, these individuals play a dominant role through their memberships and offices in enacting policies and standards and through their research in influencing our clinical practices.

Private Practice

Who is in private practice? The answer to that question is somewhat complicated. According to results of the 1985 ASHA Omnibus Survey, 9.2% of all speech-language pathologists listed private practice as their primary employment activity. But *private practice* may mean different things. Shewan (1987) reported that survey respondents included having one's own office, working in a physician's office, and holding multiple contracts in other settings (nursing homes, home health agencies, etc.) in the private-practice category. Is working for a physician "private practice"? The following definition of private practice was approved by ASHA's Legislative Council in November 1986:

A private practice is one in which a speech-language pathologist or audiologist singly or in affiliation with one or more individuals

1. has total ethical, professional, and administrative control of the practice.
2. has total financial and legal responsibility and liability for the practice.
3. is self-employed, that is, not an employee of an individual, organization, agency, or other entity providing clinical or consultative services unless also the owner of that organization or entity. (This condition will be met if the practitioner is an officer of the board of the entity and holds as much voting power as any other member of the board, even though the practitioner may not hold stock in the entity).

4. accepts referrals from multiple sources, and these referrals may include those obtained through independent contractor arrangements.

This definition may not be acceptable to all persons in the field who call themselves private practitioners, but it is the official one and is consistent with definitions of private practice in other professions.

Although some individuals have maintained private practices for decades, this segment of our field is considered to be the newest and fastest-growing practice setting. The advent of private practice in speech-language pathology has not been without controversy. Questions have been raised about speech-language pathologists as entrepreneurs. Private practitioners are, after all, in business to make money as well as to provide a needed service. The development of large speech-language pathology and audiology corporations, such as Inspeech (see Malone, 1987) has been even more controversial. Remember that most speech-language pathologists and audiologists have been salaried employees of nonprofit organizations and institutions. Many other health professionals, with whom we often want parity, have always been private practitioners. It is ironic that as we attempt to establish private practices, large numbers of physicians are become salaried employees of corporations such as health maintenance organizations (see chapter 8).

Like traditional physicians' practices, private practices in communication disorders are organized in several ways. Some persons maintain a sole proprietorship (solo practice, or a single owner who hires other practitioners); others establish partnerships (two professionals) or group practices (two or more professionals). Many practitioners form professional corporations (PCs), a legal business entity separate from the individual who owns it. These can range from small to large operations.

Referrals to private practitioners typically come from many sources including physicians, hospitals, other health professionals, community agencies, and schools. A practitioner may, of course, limit his or her particular patient population or setting. For example, you may want to work only with nursing homes and home health agencies, or see only young children. Some practitioners have formed rehabilitation agencies (RAs) or participate in comprehensive outpatient rehabilitation facilities (CORF) in order to receive payment for services rendered to Medicare beneficiaries. These are federal government designations that carry certain requirements and restrictions, including the provision of other professional services. More information about these Medicare provider types is found in chapter 8.

Is private practice for you? It is unlikely that a newly certified individual will have the experience or expertise necessary to begin a successful private practice. You may, however, wish to seek employment with an already established individual or group of practitioners. According to Shewan (1987), private practitioners, on the average, have 9.5 years of work experience, 6 more than the average ASHA member. Private practitioners also spend almost 71% of their time in clinical service delivery compared with about 59% for other ASHA members. Private practice takes a great deal of initiative. No one will be rushing to your door to sign contracts or to make appointments. You must be willing to expend a great deal of time and energy to develop and retain a clientele. If you employ other professionals and/or support staff, you will also need to develop supervisory and human resources management skills. If you want to receive payment for your services, you must learn about the third-party-payment system. The health-insurance industry is complex and ever-changing. Compliance with conditions of participation in government health programs also requires investments of time and money. For those clients who are not covered by either private or public health insurance, you will need to collect fees directly.

In order to begin a practice, as in any business venture, an individual must determine the feasibility of locating in a particular area; start-up and operating costs; procedures for managing fees, payments, and collections; the type of organizational structure desired; methods of marketing services; legal require-ments; malpractice and liability insurance needs; and other business issues. A private practitioner also needs to be knowledgeable about common business practices, business law, and administration, as well as accounting and tax require-ments. There are a variety of courses and seminars one can attend, and many business consultants are available. A list of publications and resources is provided in Appendix C for easy reference. It is by no means an exhaustive list, but the information included should be in every private practitioner's library.

In return for the independence, flexibility, and potential for higher financial gain than many salaried positions in speech-language pathology, the private practitioner faces some frustrations. Self-employed persons may have to work long hours; time out for vacations or illnesses means lost revenues; and overhead costs for materials, equipment, insurance, rent, accounting and legal services, salaries of support and other professional personnel may be high. ASHA's publication *Planning and Initiating a Private Practice in Audiology and Speech-Language Pathology* contains a list of the most common causes of private-practice failures. These causes include the following:

- lack of commitment
- inadequate fiscal planning and resources
- inappropriate facilities
- lack of business-management skills
- service offerings too restricted
- personnel difficulties
- stress-related illnesses
- personal problems

Several major private-practice trends are likely to occur in the near future.

1. Increased diversity of contracts
2. More group ownership and partnerships and corporations of mixed disciplines
3. Broader geographic bases and more multiple-location practices

4. Increased competition and more sophisticated marketing strategies
5. Increased emphasis on business-management skills

These emerging trends in private practice suggest that the larger practices will be most successful in the future. As we have discussed, the rest of the health-care industry is also moving away from fee-for-service solo practices toward large corporate medical entities.

Now that we have given you the caveats, we will also tell you that the success or failure of the trend toward private practice in the speech-language pathology and audiology professions will probably determine the course of the field in the coming years. According to Cooper (1982), "It has been suggested that one may judge how highly a professional service is valued by society by the extent to which that service is carried on by private practitioners" (p. 952). Time will tell if Cooper is right. You will be among the professionals who decide the issue.

Health Care

We have chosen to separate our discussions about working in health-care settings for the sake of order, but doing so may be misleading. Health care is a complicated business today. What you think you know about hospitals, long-term care, home-care agencies, rehabilitation facilities, and outpatient clinics today may be obsolete tomorrow. As the health-care community diversifies to meet the challenges of new payment and delivery systems, mergers, joint ventures, shared services, and integrations of services are becoming the norm. A large hospital may have a rehabilitation unit and a home health agency, sponsor a preferred provider organization (PPO), and run a large outpatient clinic. It might even own a nursing home, or at least have designated skilled-nursing beds. That means a speech-language pathologist who works for a hospital might work in any one (or all) of its units or facilities, providing different types of services to a population with an age range from birth to 100. Although that scenario may seem extreme, it is still possible.

With this varied picture in mind we provide in this section a brief introduction to clinical practice in various aspects of the health-care field.

Hospitals

Describing the "hospital experience" for speech-language pathologists is not an easy endeavor. There are general acute-care hospitals, rehabilitation institutes, children's and women's hospitals, and facilities that specialize in treating particular populations (e.g., veterans), illnesses (e.g., cancer), or parts of the body (e.g., eyes and ears). Other specialty inpatient settings include psychiatric centers, diagnostic clinics, and substance-abuse centers. Some facilities and programs are internationally known; others are small community operations. Obviously, we cannot list all the variables that may affect the clinical practice of speech-language pathology in all cases, but we can provide an introduction to some "typical" hospitals.

Let's start big: a regional rehabilitation institute. In Hospital A you will begin as a staff speech-language pathologist supervised by one of several clinical supervisors who report to the director of communicative disorders. Elaborate procedures, materials, and equipment abound. This department's approach to evaluation and treatment sometimes sets standards in the field. The program includes special subunits for augmentative communication, dysphagia, and pediatric head trauma. Several clinical research studies are always in progress. All clinicians have many opportunities to interact with rehabilitation team members; transdisciplinary treatment sessions are often shared between the speech-language pathologist and occupational therapist. People travel from all over the country to attend continuing education programs offered by the Department of Communicative Disorders and the institute's Center for Continuing Education. Sound fabulous? It is real, but there are relatively few such opportunities.

A more down-to-earth experience is represented by Hospital B, a general acute-care facility. There might be a separate department of speech-language pathology and audiology, or the services may be a part of a medical department (neurology, ENT), or a department of physical medicine. Inpatient referrals run the gamut from communication disorders associated with head and neck cancer to head injury to stroke. Table 2.2 contains examples of speech-language pathology caseloads for different units of the hospital.

TABLE 2.2
Examples of Speech-Language Pathology Caseloads in Hospitals

Unit	Possible Case Mix
Neurosurgical	Adult neurologically impaired patients, including communication disorders of aphasia, apraxia, dysarthria, dementia, confused language, and cognitive impairment. Dysphagia is also common
Shock Trauma	Neurologically impaired patients of all ages with communication disorders secondary to traumatic head injury or spinal cord injury
Coronary Care	Tracheostomy patients who may need a temporary means of communication. Also, aphasic patients secondary to cerebral ischemia or CVA
Intensive Care	Laryngectomy, CVA, shock trauma
Pediatric	Neurologically impaired children, developmental delay, voice disorders
Head and Neck Cancer or Medical/Surgical Unit	Partial or total laryngectomy, mandibulectomy, glossectomy, mechanical dysphagia
Rehabilitation	Neurologically impaired patients past the intensive-care stage

NOTE: From "Hospitals" by C. Frattali in C. Frattali and B. Cornett, 1985, *Professional affairs curriculum for communication disorders.* Unpublished manuscript.

The speech-language pathologists of Hospital B are usually responsible for five or six "billable" hours per day; that means they are expected to engage in direct patient-care activities (evaluation, treatment, counseling) or consultations for which a charge can be made. They spend the remainder of the workday keeping records, writing reports, charting in the medical record, attending case staffings, following up on referrals, and returning phone calls. Weekly or biweekly activities may include hospital grand rounds, medical department rounds, inservice programs, and rehabilitation team conferences. There are also requirements for the hospital's quality-assurance (QA) and utilization-review (UR) committees, as well as special paperwork procedures for Medicare and Medicaid patients.

As a large general hospital that wants to be competitive with other health-care-delivery systems, Hospital B is diversifying and integrating services. The speech-language pathology and audiology department is now involved in every phase of patient care, encompassing acute care, extended care, home care, and outpatient services. Some clinicians see only home-care patients, whereas others treat both inpatients and outpatients.

What about Hospital C? This facility is a community hospital in a small town. It is struggling to stay open and may soon be bought by a national for-profit hospital chain. Meanwhile, it employs no salaried speech-language pathologist but contracts with a local private practitioner. She sees inpatients on an as-needed basis. Some of those patients later come to her office for outpatient services or are referred to other facilities many miles away.

About 23% of the ASHA membership currently work in hospitals. According to the American Hospital Association (1986), hospital speech-language pathology and audiology staffs increased by more than 10% between 1983 and 1985, contrary to a national trend of hospital staff reductions. The future appears to be very bright for clinical practice in hospital settings, but there will be challenges as the entire health-care delivery system responds to cost-containment and quality-of-care issues. Health professionals will experience increased competition for patients and reimbursement dollars as well as pressure to prove the necessity for and quality of services rendered. Cooperation, skillful interprofessional relations, and careful long-range planning will be needed to assure the profession's integral role in the hospital service delivery system.

Long-Term Care

Long-term care (LTC) is the provision of health and social services to chronically ill and functionally impaired persons. A range of services is offered according to the level of care needed. Options include inpatient institutional care, day hospitals and rehabilitation centers, adult day-care programs, community group homes, and home care. Long-term-care services encompass the elderly, disabled, mentally retarded/developmentally disabled (MR/DD), mentally ill, and incarcerated populations. LTC facilities that seek Medicare and/or Medicaid reimbursement must meet certain "conditions of participation." These conditions set minimum federal and state requirements for physical environment, skilled nursing, rehabilitation, and support services in designated facilities.

The long-term-care industry is undergoing rapid change and expansion in the United States because of modifications in health-care reimbursement and demographics. There is also growing recognition that nursing homes should no longer be places for the elderly to "mark time" and that other institutions should do more than provide basic necessities for their residents. It is estimated that by the year 2020 there will be more than 60 million persons aged 65 and older (Fein, 1984). By that time, almost 13 million persons will need some form of long-term care, with 4 million requiring institutionalization.

Since the inception of Medicare's Prospective Payment System (PPS), nursing homes are receiving patients "quicker and sicker" from acute-care facilities. Nursing-home care is less costly than inpatient acute care, and long-term-care services are currently not included in PPS. Therefore, free-standing nursing facilities are becoming more interested in increasing their scope of services, especially rehabilitation. Acute-care hospitals are also developing long-term-care components, including skilled-nursing units and home-care services. As a result, the employment outlook for speech-language pathologists interested in long-term care is very promising.

Speech-language pathology services are delivered in LTC settings in a variety of ways. Only 1.6% of ASHA members work primarily in nursing homes, but many others provide services under contractual arrangements in both nursing homes and other long-term-care facilities as well as noninstitutional LTC settings. The speech-language pathologist may be a salaried employee of the facility, a private practitioner, an independent contractor, or an employee of a diversified health-care organization or other community entity that delivers services to LTC patients. A speech-language pathologist may travel to several facilities each week or work in one large facility.

In the past, national studies of nursing homes have suggested that this population is underserved with regard to rehabilitation services. That problem is diminishing as LTC facilities strive to upgrade their public image and as demand for comprehensive long-term care increases. However, speech-language-hearing professionals must continue to focus on increasing the visibility of the profession in long-term-care settings as well as develop unique services for the diverse populations served.

According to Lubinski (1981), the role of the speech-language pathologist who works in long-term-care institutions is somewhat different from that in other practice settings. Diagnostic and treatment services must be geared to very specific needs; often, traditional approaches are impossible. Innovation and creativity in every aspect of care are usually required. Additionally, the speech-language pathologist must focus a great deal of attention on the "communication-impaired environment" by identifying, assessing, modifying, or eliminating those factors that inhibit successful communication for groups as well as individual patients. One will also have to advocate for the patient's special communication needs and educate other professionals about the value of speech-language pathology services for the LTC population. Speech-language pathologists who work in psychiatric LTC institutions and those who serve the MR/DD population are especially aware of the need for advocacy, education, and collaboration with other members of the patient-care team. Prisoners constitute an underserved population for speech-language pathologists. So many opportunities exist for clinicians interested in providing services to this group. A very few professionals have developed successful communication rehabilitation programs for some of these individuals, focusing on language learning problems, factors inhibiting communicative success, and interpersonal communication problems.

Special practice settings require specific knowledge. Speech-language pathologists who work primarily with the geriatric population will want to acquire expertise in communication problems of the elderly as well as knowledge about the psychology of aging and institutional living. Other areas of interest for LTC clinicians include psychiatry, abnormal psychology, counseling, criminal justice, and advanced knowledge of communication problems associated with special populations. Appendix D contains a list of resources for professionals interested in long-term care.

We have said that long-term-care services are provided on a continuum from intensive inpatient settings to home care. Home care is discussed separately as a practice setting for speech-language pathologists because it is becoming an increasingly important health-care environment for both short-term and long-term services.

Home Care

Briefly defined, home care is the provision of health care and homemaker services in the patient's home. A team of health-care professionals works with the patient and his or her family and caregivers to restore physical, communicative, social-emotional, and other functional skills. Cost-containment efforts have promoted health-care services in settings less costly than hospitals. Consequently, the home health field is growing and thriving. Between 1974 and 1984 the number of home health visits rose from 8.2 million to 40.5 million.

Agencies that provide home health services may be proprietary or nonprofit. Medicare-certified Home Health Agencies (HHAs) must meet certain "conditions of participation." Specific services must be offered, and there are strict rules for patient eligibility. When home health services were first offered, they were sponsored primarily by visiting nurses associations (VNAs). Now, they are offered by various public and private organizations and institutions, including national companies. Many hospitals, diversifying to meet the increasing demand for alternatives to inpatient care, are also organizing home health agencies. In 1986 the top four sponsors of home-care services were: hospitals, rehabilitation facilities, for-profit companies, and private nonprofit organizations.

Speech-language pathologists whose primary employment setting is a home health agency presently comprise less than 2% of the ASHA membership, but many more practitioners probably participate in home care through private contracting or working for a hospital or other agency that offers home care in addition to other health-care services. Home care will likely be a primary speech-language pathology practice setting within the next 10 years.

As a member of the home-care team, a speech-language pathologist may perform a variety of services, including serving as the home-care team coordinator. Team membership varies, but typically a nurse, physical and occupational therapist, physician, psychologist, nutritionist, social worker, speech-language pathologist, and home health aide are involved as needed. Family members or other primary caregivers are always an integral part of the team. Collaboration and coordination of services are crucial to patient management.

What do speech-language pathologists do in the home-care setting? According to a 1981 survey conducted by Lubinski and Chapey (Lubinski, 1981), 61% of staff time is spent in treatment; 12% in diagnostic activities, 8% counseling; 5% administrative duties, and 12% travel time. In addition to providing assessment and treatment services, the speech-language pathologist also participates in team conferences, recommends referrals, provides inservice education to other professionals, completes appropriate records and reports, participates in discharge planning delivered in the home setting, evaluates the quality of services, serves as an administrator or supervisor, and conducts research studies.

The home environment is conducive to the development of creative diagnostic and treatment methods and approaches. Treatment sessions can be very natural, functional, and comfortable. The immediate relevance of goals and activities can often be observed, and the patient more easily generalizes newly learned skills in the primary setting in which they will be applied. This setting, however, is not without its challenges and frustrations.

Complaints of speech-language pathologists and other professionals who work in patients' homes may include

1. transportation problems due to time factors, weather, or vehicle malfunctions;
2. interruptions, distractions, and interference during treatment sessions;
3. lack of family motivation and commitment to the patient's rehabilitation;
4. lack of coordination of services;
5. paperwork requirements; and
6. scheduling difficulties.

Each clinician can add to or subtract from this list, depending upon his or her own experience and tolerance. Few, if any, problems are insurmountable, and the rewards usually outweigh the disadvantages. A home-care caseload can often be easily combined with nursing-home and/or clinic responsibilities so that the clinician is not always traveling. It will be interesting to observe and participate in developments in this relatively new and exciting work setting.

Hospice.   A hospice may be regarded as a specialized form of the home-care concept. The interdisciplinary team uses a holistic approach to provide support and palliative services to terminally ill patients and their families during and after the process of dying. Although most hospice programs take place in patients' homes, free-standing facilities and hospital-based units are developing rapidly. Hospice services are provided through Medicare benefits for eligible patients. Speech-language pathology services are included in the conditions of participation of Medicare-certified programs.

In this setting the goal of the speech-language pathologist is to help the patient maintain communication with family members, caregivers, and health professionals. The majority of hospice patients have long-term illnesses, such as cancer or a neurogenic disease. Patients require assistance with a variety of communication and related problems such as control of phonation/respiration, maintenance of speech intelligibility, swallowing, and cognitive/communication functions. The speech-language pathologist is also responsible for evaluating and selecting augmentative communication systems and devices for patients, as well as training and maintaining the patient's, family's, and professionals' use of such systems. Counseling is as much a part of the speech-language pathologist's role as direct treatment.

Working in a hospice may be rewarding for persons who are emotionally mature and want to participate in a very special kind of patient care: maintaining, adapting, and modifying the patient's communication mode to fit his or her changing skills, needs, and overall environment. Communication is our most human characteristic, and it is crucial that dying patients and their families be able to express their needs and feelings throughout the course of illness.

Community Clinics

Community clinic is a generic term that covers the gamut of public and private nonprofit organizations that provide speech-language-hearing and other services to community residents. These clinics may be operated by national and local associations or societies (e.g., Easter Seal Society, United Cerebral Palsy), public health departments, hospitals, and other private or government programs. They are funded by tax dollars, United Way, and other fund-raising groups, and fee-for-service (usually based on ability to pay). Most clinics are governed by a board of directors that hires executive staff to administer the programs.

Speech-language pathologists who work in community clinic settings are involved in a wide variety of activities and services, including prevention and public education, screenings, diagnosis and treatment of communication disorders, counseling, inservice education, and consultation. There are also many opportunities for clinicians interested in supervisory and administrative work. Depending upon the type of clinic, patient caseloads can be highly specialized or encompass the entire scope of communication disorders and age groups. Some community clinics have contracts with other facilities and programs, so that speech-language pathology staff may provide services to home-care, nursing-home, hospital, and public school patients and clients as well as persons who come to the clinic.

Salaries and benefits vary with the agency, but in general, salaries are lower than those in other work settings, with the exception of public schools. Community clinics often depend upon "soft" funding, that is, grant monies, contributions, and percentages of communitywide fund-raising campaigns for a substantial portion of the clinic budget. Thus, administrators must constantly be concerned about maintaining staff positions, services, and facilities. Community clinics are competing with private practitioners, hospital outpatient departments, health maintenance organizations, and other new health programs. Cutbacks in government and community funding also mean that community clinics will be seeking to develop new services and different ways of packaging and delivering existing services. Strong community support and a broad referral base will be important advantages to clinics in funding efforts.

Challenges to community-based speech-language-hearing programs may actually provide more opportunities for clinicians and administrators who want to expand, modify, and coordinate services in creative ways. Speech-language pathologists who enjoy this type of position appreciate the opportunities to interact with other professionals and citizens' groups. A clinician may also specialize in communication disorders of specific populations in certain agencies or become a generalist in the truest sense of the word in other situations. Community clinics offer speech-language pathologists a grass-roots approach to professional practice that many clinicians would not trade for anything else.

HMOs and PPOs

The so-called alternative health-care-delivery system is quickly becoming an integral part of the mainstream of health services in this country. Health maintenance organizations (HMOs) and preferred provider organizations (PPOs) are considered alternatives to the traditional fee-for-service system because they present different mechanisms for organizing both payment and delivery of services. HMOs act both as insurers and providers of care. Enrollees (patients) receive a range of services for a prepaid fee. PPOs are sponsored by providers, entrepreneurs, or purchasers who contract with a designated panel of health professionals to provide services to a defined population according to a negotiated fee schedule. Both types of organizations purport to reduce health-care costs and promote quality by coordinating patient access to and utilization of health services. The goal is to spend money on keeping the patient well and out of hospitals. Chapter 8 contains more detailed information about these health-care systems.

Speech-language pathologists who currently practice in these settings are pioneers. Their experiences will set the stage for defining, expanding, and refining our professional roles in these organizations. At this point, it is difficult to describe accurately the clinical practice of speech-language pathology in HMOs, but some data are available. According to the Group Health Association of America, a trade association for many of the nation's HMOs, over 90% of their member HMOs cover at least some speech-language pathology or audiology services. These services may require copayments by the enrollees, and coverage is often restricted to a certain number of sessions and for limited types of communication disorders (usually related to a medical condition).

A survey we conducted more than a year ago (Cornett & Chabon, 1986) queried medical directors of approximately 50 HMOs about various policies regarding speech-language pathology services. Results suggested that most speech-language pathology services are provided through contractual arrangements or informal referral arrangements. Only 12% of the respondents indicated that they employed salaried speech-language pathologists. The same survey revealed that a majority of HMOs restrict rehabilitation services to two months because that is the guideline stated in federal regulations pertaining to the HMO act of 1973.

Our profession is challenged to develop new service delivery mechanisms in HMOs while we also attempt to educate administrators and primary-care personnel about some of our patients' needs for longer term rehabilitation. We will need to produce data for HMOs on expected lengths of treatment for specific communication disorders and provide prognostic indicators. Unrestricted, unmonitored service delivery is not consistent with the HMO concept. Therefore, the successful HMO speech-language pathologist will be able to meet these data needs as well as provide such services as screenings, health-promotion and prevention programs, and different approaches to assessment and treatment in conjunction with other HMO providers.

Another interesting option for speech-language pathologists and audiologists in private practice is to organize an independent practice association (IPA). An IPA is a form of HMO in which independent practitioners form a contractual alliance with each other and with a staff- or group-model HMO to provide specified services to the HMO's enrollees. In this way, speech-language-hearing professionals can offer an array of services over a broader geographic base. Quality review mechanisms are also likely to be more feasible, and there is more power in numbers.

PPOs achieve their cost savings through fee negotiation and discounting, as well as strong utilization review. Selective contracting with cost-effective, efficient providers is the key in this setting. There is no reason why speech-language pathologists and audiologists cannot become a part of the PPO system. But, it will require cooperation among private practitioners, clinics, and other facilities and a peer-review mechanism to promote quality services while controlling for overutilization.

It is very likely that many of the readers of this book will become involved with HMOs, PPOs, and other new service delivery systems. These organizations are expanding the scope of their services by enrolling Medicare beneficiaries and by recognizing the need to change the focus of their services from acute-care to include home health and other longer term health-care services. These developments are encouraging for rehabilitation professionals, but we will have to be assertive, creative, flexible, and accountable in order to establish ourselves better in these settings.

■ SUMMARY

We have presented vignettes about the places and programs in which speech-language pathologists work and have provided a picture of each practice setting as well as facts and figures. We wanted to share with you, our readers, what we view as the most important and interesting aspects—both the positive and the frustrating—of each place or program. We hope this information will stimulate your curiosity about one or several employment possibilities. Opportunities for clinical practice are increasing, and the number of settings in which we work continues to expand. Whatever you decide, we encourage you to concentrate on developing your knowledge, skills, and commitment to the field and to the needs of the communicatively handicapped so that, wherever you work, the title *speech-language pathologist* will mean *excellence*.

ACTIVITIES

1. Identify at least three settings in which you might like to work. Provide your reasons for choosing these.

2. Prepare a sample resume that includes all relevant clinical and academic background and your employment history.

3. Considering your current career plans, describe other experiences/coursework you wish to complete before graduation.

4. Contact a local speech and hearing facility and request a copy of a job description for an entry-level speech-language pathologist.

5. Interview speech-language pathologists in at least two different clinical practice settings to determine what they see as the primary advantages/disadvantages of the setting
   a. to the clients served,
   b. to the speech-language pathologists employed there,
   c. to the students engaged in practicum there.

6. Compare results obtained in activity 5 with responses to a second interview conducted with student clinicians who have completed or are in the process of completing practicum experiences in the same or similar clinicial sites.

7. With another graduate student clinician conduct a role play of a job interview for a speech-language pathologist or audiologist in one of the employment settings identified in the chapter.

8. Identify at least two of your traits, skills, or experiences that would make you especially well qualified to work in the setting of your choice.

9. Poll your classmates to determine the most/least popular settings for future employment.

10. Identify the settings in which the members of your current state or national professional associations' executive board members are employed.

REFERENCES

American Hospital Association (1986). *Effects of the Medicare prospective pricing system on hospital staffing* (p. 17). Chicago, IL: AHA.

Arnett, R., McKusick, D., Sonnefeld, S., & Corwell, C. (1985). Projections of health care spending to 1990. *Health Care Financing Review, 7*(3), 1–36.

ASHA. *Omnibus survey.* (1984). Rockville, MD.

ASHA (1985). *Services in home health settings* [Teleconference Cassettes]. Rockville, MD.

ASHA Committee on Language, Speech, and Hearing Services in the Schools. (1984). Recommended service delivery models and caseload sizes for speech-language pathology services in the schools. *Asha, 26*(4), 53–58.

ASHA Committee on Supervision and Council on Professional Standards. (1982). Minimum qualifications for supervisors and suggested competencies for effective clinical supervision. *Asha, 24*(5), 339–342.

ASHA Committee on Supervision. (1985). Clinical supervision in speech-language pathology and audiology. *Asha, 27*(6), 57–60.

ASHA Committee on Supervision. (1982). Suggested competencies for effective supervision. *Asha, 24*(12), 1021–1023.

Cole, P. (1986). I want to shape my own future. How about you? *Asha, 28*(9), 41–42.

Cooper, E. (1982). The state of the profession and what to do about it: One lover's quarrel. *Asha, 24*(11), 931–934.

Cornett, B., & Chabon, S. (1986, November). Speech-language pathologists: Winners or losers in the health care revolution? Paper presented at the meeting of the American Speech-Language-Hearing Association, Detroit, MI.

Digest of Education Statistics. (1983–1984). Reprinted in "The Communicator," *Language News in Special Education, 1*(2). Phoenix, AZ: Syndactics.

Education of the Handicapped Act becomes law. (1986). *Government Affairs Review, 7*(4), 427–436.

Eger, D. L. (1986). *School issues: Gaining support for your program.* [Teleconference Manual]. Rockville, MD: ASHA.

Evashwick, C. (1987). Home health care: Current trends and future opportunities. In N. Goldfield & S. Goldsmith (Eds.), *Alternative delivery systems* (pp. 5–18). Rockville, MD: Aspen Systems.

Fein, D. (1984). On aging. *Asha, 26*(8), 25.

Flower, R. M. (1984). *Delivery of speech-language pathology and audiology services.* Baltimore, MD: Williams & Wilkins.

Frassinelli, L., Superior, K., & Meyers, J. (1983). A consultation model for speech and language intervention. *Asha, 25*(11), 25–30.

Hardick, E. J., & Oyer, H. J. (1987) Administration of speech-language hearing programs within the university setting. In H. J. Oyer (Ed.), *Administration of programs in speech-language pathology and audiology.* Englewood Cliffs, NJ: Prentice-Hall.

Hyman, C. (1986). The 1985 omnibus survey: Implications for strategic planning. *Asha, 28*(4), 19–22.

———. (1987, July). *Demographic profile of the ASHA membership.* Rockville, MD: ASHA.

Jones, S., & Healey, W. C. (1973). Phase 1: Recommendations for state departments of education in implementing comprehensive regulations for language, speech, and hearing services in schools. *Project Upgrade: Model regulations for school language, speech, and hearing programs and services.* Washington, DC: ASHA.

Kamara, C. (1986). ASHA's professional practices activities. *Asha, 28*(9), 25–28.

Larkins, P. (1986). The challenges ahead for the practice of speech-language pathology. *Asha, 28*(9), 29–30.

Light, D. W, Mardsen, L. R., & Corl, T. C. (1973). *The impact of the academic revolution on faculty careers.* Washington, DC: American Association for Higher Education.

Lubinski, R. (1981). Environmental language intervention. In R. Chapey (Ed.), *Language intervention strategies in adult aphasia* (pp. 223–245). Baltimore, MD: Williams & Wilkins.

Malone, R. (1987). InSpeech: inbusiness, inspired. *Asha, 29*(1), 35–39.

Maxwell, S. (1986). Public school caucus: A professional partnership. *Asha, 28*(5), 26.

Minifie, F. (1983). ASHA is planning for the future. *Asha, 25*(5), 29–30.

Neidecker, E. A. (1980). *School programs in speech-language: organization and management.* Englewood Cliffs, NJ: Prentice-Hall.

Pickering, M. (1981). Consulting with the classroom teacher to promote language acquisition and usage. *Topics in Learning and Learning Disabilities, 1*(2), 41–46.

Sarnecky, E. (1987). Speech-language pathology and audiology: A profession that lets you be what you want to be. *Career and Higher Education News, 1,* 3.

Shewan, C. (1987). Who is a private practitioner? *Asha, 29*(1), 59.

Silverman, F. (1983). *Legal aspects of speech-language pathology: An overview of law for clinicians, researchers, and teachers.* Englewood Cliffs, NJ: Prentice-Hall.

Sommers, R. K. & Hatton, M. E. (1985). Establishing the therapy program: Case finding, case selection, and caseload. In R. J. Van Hattum (Ed.), *Organization of speech-language services in schools.* San Diego, CA: College-Hill Press.

Staff. (1986). From pre-school to high school speech-language-hearing services in the public schools: A class act. *Asha, 28*(5), 18–21.

Tanner, D. (1980). Loss and grief: Implications for the speech-language pathologist and audiologist. *Asha, 22*(10), 916–928.

Taylor, J. S. (1981). *Speech-language pathology services in the schools.* New York: Grune & Stratton.

Wilson, L. (1942). *The academic man. A study in the sociology of a profession.* New York: Oxford University Press.

CHAPTER THREE

Platitudes on Attitudes

INTRODUCTION

"If I only had a brain . . . If I only had a heart . . . If I only had the nerve," sang the Scarecrow, the Tin Man, and the Cowardly Lion, respectively, in Harold Arlen and E. Y. Harburg's song from *The Wizard of Oz*. These characters' wishes parallel three attitudes that are central to high-quality clinical services. The first is a *scientific attitude*, which represents the theoretical knowledge and scientific data base, the *brain* with which to structure and develop our clinical methods. Its importance can be illustrated by the many technical advances and scholarly achievements that have modified and strengthened our understanding of normal and disordered communication.

The second, a *therapeutic attitude*, refers to our caring and compassionate behaviors, the *heart* and soul that we pour into our clinical endeavors. These interpersonal skills are essential in creating an atmosphere in which change can occur.

The third is a *professional attitude*, which encompasses the substantive aspects, occupational values, and economic principles of clinical work. These traits give us the courage, or *nerve,* to define our professional roles.

Sarason (1985), in his seminal book about clinical practice, asserts that "what the clinician experiences after finishing training is a continuation of an attitude, of a way of structuring professional life, that was absorbed before entering practice" (p. 175). Sarason poses the following questions: "What kind of person do we want the clinician to be, and how do we help such a person become that?'' (p. 182). We wish to instill in the student clinician an understanding of the importance of scientific commitment, caring and compassion, and professionalism that will evolve and grow stronger throughout his or her professional career. We firmly believe that we can best serve our clients only when these three attitudes—scientific, therapeutic, and professional—coexist.

THE SCIENTIFIC ATTITUDE IN CLINICAL PRACTICE

> I'd unravel ev'ry riddle
> for any individle
> In trouble or in pain . . .
> If I only had a brain.
> —Harburg & Arlen, ''If I Only Had a Brain''

When we think about science, many of us conjure up visions of bubbling test tubes, absent-minded professors, frog dissections, and Dr. Frankenstein's monster. When we are less imaginative, but more intimidated, we may consider science a ''lofty endeavor performed by individuals who do not necessarily walk on the same ground as the common man'' (Prutting, 1983, p. 248). Should science really be so frightening? *Webster's Unabridged Dictionary* defines *science* as ''systematized knowledge derived from observation, study, and experimentation.'' According to Hildebrand (1957), science has two components: *content* and *enterprise*. Content refers to the technical and procedural aspects of classifying knowledge, whereas enterprise is the creativity, intuition, educated guesses, and spirit of inquiry and discovery involved in the research process. Enterprise prevents content from becoming too dry and laborious, from taking the fun and passion out of observing the world.

Science is at the heart of the discipline of human communication sciences and disorders. The American Speech-Language-Hearing Association states in its bylaws that among the purposes of the association are the basic scientific study of the processes of human communication, the promotion of the investigation and prevention of communication disorders, and the exchange and dissemination of information related to these goals. Patricia Cole (1987), in her first official interview as ASHA president, observed that ''our future is closely tied to the strength of our science and research base. If we don't have that base, then we are going to be technicians who must rely on other professions to tell us what to do'' (p. 26). Many clinicians may conclude that Cole's statement is meant for the researchers of the field of speech-language pathology and audiology, those who ''do'' science in universities or other research centers. Only 1.3% of ASHA members consider research to be their primary employment activity; 4.4% are primarily college or university professors. About 70% of ASHA members are direct clinical service providers. Unfortunately, many of these practitioners may say that the science of the profession should be left to the scientists; clinicians should only provide clinical services. Were that to happen, the profession would indeed be far less than scientific.

In fact, there has been considerable controversy about the scientific basis for the profession of speech-language pathology and audiology, especially as science relates to clinical practice. Kamhi (1984) argues that clinicians should function as "clinical scientists" throughout the diagnostic and therapeutic process. He contends that many clinicians view science as necessary only in research:

> Some no doubt, view science as being rigid and inflexible where, in fact, the opposite is closer to the truth. By gathering clinical data and formulating and testing hypotheses based on these data, the clinician ensures that the clinical process remains flexible and attuned to the client's changing needs. In this way diagnosis becomes an ongoing process rather than a one-time occurrence at the initial evaluation. (p. 227)

Kamhi maintains that clinical work and research involve similar problem-solving skills, including the formulation, testing, confirmation or refutation, and reformulation of hypotheses. Ringel (1972) also believes that clinical practice and research share many of the same goals and procedures. He developed a very useful description of the relationship between research and clinical activities, as outlined in Figure 3.1.

Although Hegde (1985) agrees that there are striking similarities between scientific and clinical activities, he is careful to point out the distinctions between routine clinical work and scientific research, stating that "the difference lies in the amount of care taken to rule out the influence of extraneous independent variables" (p. 25). He suggests the following:

> The clinical researcher may wish to isolate the original or the maintaining cause of a given disorder, or an effective treatment for it. In achieving these goals, however, the clinical researcher must follow the same procedures the scientist follows. Just like the scientist, the clinical researcher rules out extraneous independent variables, manipulates a specific independent variable (treatment), produces changes in a dependent variable (communicative behavior or disorder), and thus establishes a cause-and-effect relation between the treatment and client behavior. (p. 26)

Hegde argues that in order to document the effectiveness of treatment, we must rule out the influence of other variables. The fact that a client/patient may improve during the course of treatment does not mean that the improvement was a direct result of intervention. Controlled clinical research must be conducted in order to validate those procedures we believe are effective.

The single-subject research design has been suggested by a number of authors as an excellent clinical research tool for documenting treatment effectiveness; comparing various treatment methods; assessing client management strategies such as group versus individual sessions; and evaluating frequency, intensity, and duration of treatment (Barlow & Hersen, 1984; Bauer, 1985; Flower, 1984; Hegde, 1985; Kent & Fair, 1985; McReynolds & Kearns, 1982). The purpose of the single-subject design is to isolate cause-and-effect relationships. An independent

---

FIGURE 3.1 AN APPROACH TO TREATMENT AND RESEARCH ACTIVITIES

A. Diagnostic Procedure (Definition of Problem)

1. Is the disorder (research problem) clearly stated as a single issue or a series of subordinate but related dysfunctions (problems)?
2. Is the disorder (research problem) isolated and analyzed logically; use of proper tests?
3. Are there adequate definitions of significant terms used in defining the problem?
4. Is adequate use made of previous observations and test results (previous research)?

B. Treatment Rationale (The Working Hypothesis)

1. Is the treatment (hypothesis) clearly stated and pertinent to the solution of the problem?
   a. Does the formulation of the theory (hypothesis) reflect an adequate understanding of the problem?
   b. Does the general approach to development of therapy (hypothesis) reflect an objective attitude.
2. Is the presentation of the method and design of the therapeutic program (research) such that it can be duplicated and continued by other clinicians (researchers)?

C. Evaluation of Progress (The Analysis)

1. Is there adequate proof of the validity of your therapeutic approach (the data)?
2. Are the methods of evaluating therapeutic gains (data) adequate and appropriate?
3. Are the inferences drawn from the therapy evaluation (data analysis) clear, sound, and appropriately limited?

D. The Result (Conclusions)

1. Does the conclusion provide new insights, establish the validity of the therapeutic (research) procedures, or verify the conclusions of previous clinicians (researchers)?
2. Does the conclusion bear a reasonable relationship to other known facts?
3. Does the conclusion point toward further clinical practice (research) development?

E. Case Report (Publication)

Is the patient (research) described in a fashion such that other professionals can evaluate your progress and continue the treatment (research)?

NOTE: From "The Clinician and the Researcher: An Artificial Dichotomy" by R. Ringel, 1972, *Asha*, 14(7), pp. 351–353. Copyright 1972 by R. Ringel. Reprinted by permission.

variable is systematically manipulated to determine specific effects of the independent variable on dependent variables. Single-subject research, also called the within-subject strategy, is particularly suited to the needs of clinicians because there is no need to meet the requirements of traditional between-groups strategies. For an extended discussion of both types of research see Hegde (1985).

Some of our leaders have observed that the basic science of the discipline of human communication sciences and disorders is not yet adequate because we have not developed unique theories and thus become an "autonomous science"

(Ringel, Trachtman, & Prutting, 1984). Others (Siegel & Ingham, 1987) believe that the discipline of communication sciences and disorders is not less scientific merely because it shares theories, models, methods, and concepts with the larger community of behavioral science. Siegel and Ingham (1987) refer to speech-language pathologists and audiologists as "behavioral scientists with a special focus" (p. 100). We are unique as practitioners because we are devoted to the communicatively handicapped, but as scientists we are "partners in behavioral science, with equal access to the paradigms, theories, methods and controversies that plague and energize all behavioral sciences" (p. 101).

Clinicians have the very challenging task of deciphering science and incorporating research findings into everyday clinical work. They must learn to be careful consumers of research as well as initiators of clinical studies. According to Kent (1985), the scientific clinician's four primary goals are to (1) learn about new research discoveries; (2) apply selected research information to clinical practice; (3) evaluate empirically his or her own intervention; and (4) conduct research in the clinical setting. Siegel and Ingham (1987) suggest that theory, research, and experience are all important sources of knowledge and methods and contribute to the clinician's overall skill. Speech-language pathologists and audiologists who have a scientific orientation or attitude toward clinical practice balance theory, research, and daily experiences. The scientific clinician is skeptical—about theory as well as practice.

The core of a scientific attitude is *curiosity*. We must always be asking questions—questions about our purposes, goals, objectives, therapy methods, and research designs. Richard Flower, former ASHA president, titled his presidential address "Asking Questions" (1985). His points offer a fitting conclusion to this discussion:

> Honesty demands that we own up to our bewilderment . . . about the nature of human communication and its disorders . . . about treatment . . . about how services should be delivered and who should deliver those services and how much they should be prepared. Like all bewildered people, we ask many questions and ask them over and over again. . . . So long as we continue to ask questions we are honest, alert, alive and in good health, no matter how bewildered. A traditional toast proclaims "To life!" However redundant, I would add, "To bewilderment!" I can think of no more suitable salute to this discipline, to this profession and to this association. (p. 25)

And, we will add, To science!

THE THERAPEUTIC ATTITUDE IN CLINICAL PRACTICE

> I'd be tender, I'd be gentle
> And awful sentimental
> Regarding love and art . . .
> If I only had a heart.
> —Harburg & Arlen, "If I Only Had a Brain"

While writing this section we received a call from the mother of a child whom we had known in our clinic for more than five years. She opened the conversation by apologizing for the need to make the call, and, sounding upset, said that she had heard from the student clinician assigned to work with her son. She said that she recognized that this might be just a petty complaint but that the student who was calling to schedule therapy sessions for the term had specified only one time with no alternatives. The mother questioned the clinician about other possible openings and mentioned she had understood that the therapy time would remain the same as the one she had had in previous academic terms. She perceived a reaction of irritation and impatience and was informed that the student had already registered for classes, contacted all her other clients, and accepted a part-time job as a salesclerk and thus only had the one time available. The parent, left with no other choice, agreed to this arrangement, and then spent several hours trying to reschedule cub scouts, soccer, a carpool, and babysitting. Shortly thereafter, the student called again, this time to report that she was required to stay later than planned at her outside placement and would need to change the day of therapy. The mother, who in retelling this story grew increasingly angry, stated, "She made me feel that we are not at all important to her."

A few years ago while teaching a course in diagnostic procedures, we conducted a series of role-playing exercises. One of these involved interviewing a preschooler's parents, who disagreed about whether their child was stuttering or just passing through a stage of normal disfluency. A student who was in the fourth term of graduate school played the clinician, who was to reconcile the parents' views in terms of the reality of the situation and to defuse their arguing. Following the role play, the student said, "You know, since I have never worked with a stutterer, I have not had an opportunity to really use my interviewing skills before this." By the term *interviewing skills* she was referring to such behaviors as attending to the speaker, listening to feelings, and accepting feelings. Perhaps we should have been gratified that she realized the importance of these skills in the relationship between stutterer and therapist, but we weren't. Rather, we were concerned that a bright, well-motivated, and committed graduate student clinician was not aware that these actions of caring and concern are applicable to all clients.

We share these anecdotes because they reflect some of the difficulties in clinical work today. As we have each been involved in the clinical education of speech-language pathologists for many years, we have observed unprecedented growth in the profession's information base as evidenced in course offerings and scope of practice. The use of technology to resolve clinical problems has heightened, and the emphasis on technical skills and scientific precision has increased. However, surprisingly little attention has been paid to the emotional and social needs of those we serve. Although the quality of care in speech-language pathology has received a great deal of consideration, the quality of caring in our field has been given much less thought.

Frederic Darley (1985), in his address to the Council of Graduate Programs in Communication Sciences and Disorders about the status of clinical education, posed the following questions:

Are we making an effort to teach the therapeutic attitude? Do we consider the student's capacity to empathize? Do we show students how to relate non-defensively and insightfully? How to get inside the skins and heads of their patients? How to put up with them? How to behave? How to act—so as to facilitate improvement and improve character? (p. 11)

Darley (1985) notes that individuals who seek a career in speech-language pathology are prompted by a desire to help others. His statement suggests that individuals are "called" to speech-language pathology because it provides an opportunity to use special interests and abilities to serve others. Darley believes student clinicians are thus motivated "not just to find a career, earn a degree, get a job, make money, invest it profitably and get security, but rather to get involved, find their identity by hooking up with other people, share themselves and engage in work that involves commitment" (p. 12). He urges those of us who teach to imbue a therapeutic attitude in our students. Yet, as Sarason (1985) reports, graduate instruction in the health-care fields often fails to prepare clinicians to be caring and compassionate.

When one considers how clinicians are educated, it becomes readily apparent that schools emphasize the origins and patterns of specific communication problems. Typically, students are required to complete a certain number of disorder courses and obtain clinical experience in each of these distinct areas. There is very little focus in the academic curriculum on issues that relate to the interpersonal qualities involved in the provision of a clinical service (e.g., interpersonal communication, family counseling). A survey of 134 Educational Standards Board–accredited audiology and speech-language pathology programs revealed varied emphasis placed on and importance attached to counseling experiences. An additional finding was that graduate students often get a background in counseling theory and techniques only if they choose to do so (McCarthy, Culpepper, & Lucks, 1986).

Today, the increased diversification of the clinical population for whom we are responsible has resulted in an "information explosion." The fallout is reflected in the creation of numerous subspecialties in our field and the practical problem of what can reasonably be included in one and a half to two years of graduate school. It seems unlikely that programs of graduate study will lengthen to accommodate these new academic interests. What is probable, however, is that issues that are not viewed as central to the preparation of budding clinicians will be set aside. Programs that are already accused of failing to train clinicians to be caring and compassionate people will be further compromised in their efforts to address the dynamics of the clinical interaction. Perhaps one hope is that peer review and public scrutiny of our professional services will be incentives for us to focus our energies on fostering a therapeutic conscience.

There have been a disturbing number of accounts in the recent academic and lay literature that bemoan the absence of caring and compassionate attitudes from different groups of clinicians, but primarily physicians (Eisenstadt, 1972; Elliot, 1984; Krupat, 1986; Sarason, 1985; Shorter, 1985; Switzer, 1985). Sarason

(1985) summarized the findings of an unpublished study that examined the qualities parents of retarded children perceive as most helpful and least helpful in service providers. The most helpful professionals were "typically recalled as being 'interested,' 'concerned,' 'understanding,' and 'sensitive'," while the least helpful professionals were described as " 'discouraging,' 'insensitive,' 'cold,' and 'businesslike' " (pp. 100–101).

These parents' reactions have implications for the state of the art in our own field. It is unlikely that any of us intends to be insensitive or cold. We may view ourselves as effective communicators of empathy and concern, yet we may be perceived as uncaring. Although the high priority given to science and technology in our education and our clinical practices may account for some of the neglect of the clinician-client relationship, it neither sufficiently explains nor justifies it.

We have entered an era in which public and private third-party payors contract and pay for our services. They have imposed constraints on our time and perhaps on the nature and duration of our clinical interactions. Clinicians are becoming businesspersons. Many of us work for large bureaucratic organizations. We must now identify the proportion of our time that is billable. We can charge for time spent in administering tests and using clearly defined therapy procedures. Insurance companies will pay us whether or not these services are rendered with empathy and sensitivity. The reality is that we are asked to satisfy our clients' minimal needs at the lowest possible costs (Sarason, 1985).

As speech-language pathologists, we face another, perhaps in some ways unique, challenge. We are rarely the first professionals consulted when a communication problem is suspected. Usually a family turns first to a physician or sometimes a teacher with a question about speech, language, or hearing. The attention and caring these families receive and the amount of time they spend in seeking answers to their questions may affect the way they approach our clinical encounters. Unfortunately, the period between their first awareness of a communication difficulty and the time that a diagnosis is made or therapy is initiated can be emotionally draining and leave parents feeling frustrated, angry, and skeptical. Although the speech-language pathologist is not responsible for these feelings, a defensive or insensitive stance may contribute to or fail to reduce the client's initial misgivings.

In his description of the doctor-patient relationship, Shorter (1985) asserts that physicians have become "much more disease-oriented" and "less patient-oriented."

> Being disease-oriented means that you, the doctor, basically believe the patient has some kind of physical disease, the result perhaps of the invasion of a micro-organism (such as a cold) or of a degenerative process (such as osteoarthritis), and that you believe your job as a doctor is to diagnose and appropriately treat that disease. Therefore, encounters with disease-oriented doctors are likely to lack, for the patient, a certain human dimension. Such doctors tend to be perfunctory in history-taking (not believing the "history of the illness" to be all that revealing); to be concerned principally with gathering diagnostic data and interpreting it with specialists; and to evidence little personal interest in the patient. It is not that they are disinterested

in patients and their personal problems. It is just that there is no medical need to show interest. (p. 23)

Similarly, there is a risk that we as speech-language pathologists may be neglecting our clients as whole persons while we meticulously analyze (with the help of a computer) their articulation, count and describe their language forms and lexical selections, and time their rate and fluency of speech. Concern for the whole person with communication problems was well stated in the Hippocratic Oath proposed by West (1961) for our profession, as shown in the accompanying box.

HIPPOCRATIC OATH

These things we each declare, and jointly we all affirm:

The speech of the children of man is our interest; and the communication of man is our concern. We seek out those who are halting in speech; and we offer help to those whose ears have been confused by disease. Life without speech is empty; and life devoid of communication is scarcely better than death. Therefore the duty we owe is sacred; and our calling is gravely important. We have reverence for humanity, whom we serve, and deference for the men, women, and children whom we aid. Out of this deference grows our ethos; and from our reverence stems our professional morality. No personal advantage to us will ever lessen our concern for our pupils or patients, and no selfish consideration will ever color our advice or our instruction. What we need to know of the lives and personal affairs of our pupils and patients we will ask, but that only; and that which we learn we shall guard as a sacred trust of confidence. We shall ever revere those who instructed us in the arts of our profession; and insofar as we attempt to pass on the instruction we received we will so teach as to be worthy of the respect of our students. We will have no proprietary secrets of science or of arts; but whatever seems to us to be helpful to our pupils or patients we will freely transmit to our colleagues in the profession. We will join and support organizations in which those in our profession may commune as brothers and sisters; and in which helpful ideas may be exchanged and discussed. We will conduct our professional lives so that our colleagues will be proud to recognize us as members of their profession; and in our private lives so will we live that the public picture of our profession will be one of honor and dignity. In our relations colleague to colleague, instructor to student, clinician to patient, or teacher to pupil, we will treat all persons alike irrespective of race or relation.

These things we promise in the name of the most precious thing on earth: Humanity.

NOTE: From ''To Our New Members—*Ave et Vale*'' by R. West, 1961, *Asha,* 3(1)8.

Although these Hippocratic ideals were established years ago, it is not too late for each of us to retake these vows. As Francis Peabody, a professor at Harvard University, noted, "One of the essential qualities of the clinician is interest in humanity, for the secret of the care of the patient is in caring for the patient" (Krupat, 1986, pp. 26).

To caring!

THE PROFESSIONAL ATTITUDE IN CLINICAL PRACTICE

> But I could show my prowess,
> Be a lion, not a mowess,
> If I only had the nerve.
> —Harburg & Arlen, "If I Only Had a Brain"

I remember the student who confided to her client as she prepared to administer a series of test probes, "This is the first time I have ever used these tests, and I'm a little nervous." I also recall the student who abruptly closed an exit interview with a client by stating, "Well, I'd love to continue chatting with you, but I have an exam tonight and I need to go study." These examples suggest an attitude that may exist in student-client relationships. Do students act and respond in a manner consistent with their student status, or are their actions defined by their sense of professionalism? Is it possible for a student to have a professional attitude?

In our view, students can and in fact must convey a professional attitude throughout their clinical work if they are to assume roles as student clinicians. We recognize that students regard themselves primarily as students, and we understand that professionalism will develop and change over time. However, we believe that in any clinical interaction the clinician (even in the case of a student clinician), by accepting the responsibility of modifying the behavior of another individual, has entered a professional relationship and must, therefore, think and act accordingly.

What does it mean to be a *professional*? Perhaps both very little and a great deal. The term has evolved to the point that we commonly use it to identify diverse occupational groups as well as the so-called established professions of law, medicine, and the ministry. Professionalism is not always viewed positively; and the term is open to broad, inconsistent, and vague interpretations and is difficult to operationalize. As Moore (1970) asserts, however, "To have one's occupational conduct judged as professional is highly regarded in all post-industrial societies and in at least the modernizing sectors of others" (p. 3).

There are a number of qualities that capture for us the essence of a professional attitude. For purposes of discussion we have separated these as follows:

- *Expertise:* Includes the requisite knowledge and specialized skills and techniques often attested to by educational and certification requirements.
- *Professional Norms:* include codes of professional conduct and clinical accountability.
- *Professional Identity:* deals with issues of collegiality and professional memberships.
- *Legal Identity:* addresses those state licensure laws that regulate professional practice.
- *Business Acumen:* focuses on management and financial aspects of professional practice.
- *Personal Traits:* relate to one's professional style.

Expertise

The ability to present oneself as a professional and feel confident in the role assumes some specialized knowledge and training. The specific educational and clinical content required for professional initiation may vary over time and to some extent with the individual and the educational institution. In describing the curricula of professional schools, Moore (1970) suggests that they "always entail an irrational mixture of several components!"

1. What the professor learned, which is necessarily a collegiate generation earlier and usually a full biological generation gone into antiquity.
2. What the qualifying (and certifying) authorities think should be known; for a variety of not very subtle reasons, the persons serving on review or certifying committees are likely to represent a full biological generation—or more—in ascendancy over the new aspirants.
3. What the "new revolutionaries" on the professional school faculty think is appropriate for the training of future professionals. (p. 74)

ASHA has outlined the qualifications for entry into the practice of speech-language pathology and audiology in its Certificate of Clinical Competence. Certification is awarded to those individuals who meet educational and clinical requirements, complete the equivalent of nine months of full-time professional experience, and successfully pass a national examination. For complete information about the general curricula and specific courses currently needed to qualify for certification, refer to the current *Membership and Certification Handbook*, which can be obtained by writing to the American Speech-Language-Hearing Association.

State certification of public school clinicians is also common. There is some inconsistency in and much debate about the educational and clinical requirements for school certification from state to state. Those interested in employment within the schools should contact their state education agency for specific information about credentialing requirements.

Can an individual who has not satisfied the substantive criteria of professionalism perform with an attitude of professionalism? Our answer is an unconditional yes or at least a qualified maybe. Through our involvement in the clinical education of graduate students we have observed a number of our students respond in a manner that reflects knowledge and preparation. Their preparedness might be based on hours of independent reading, planning, and/or consultation with the supervisor for a session or a number of sessions. Students have the advantage of immediate access to current information about the field and have the opportunity to apply that information while it is fresh. The student responsible for a case must be aware of areas of competency and deficiency relative to that case in order to assure quality service. Whether the clinician has received a master's degree, has earned certification, or has just begun a graduate program, he or she is only in the midst of becoming educated. As Moore (1970) notes,

> The self-confidence that professionals display is either a pretense or a mark of self-delusion. If a little learning is a dangerous thing, then most of us must live with virtually ubiquitous danger, for most of us do have a little, and the great learning of men of knowledge is still paltry, and still dangerous. (p. 243)

Clinicians should become familiar with the particular individual to be helped and the theoretical issues surrounding that individual's problem(s) in order to feel professional and act professionally. For, as Darley (1985) so aptly pointed out, "We still have to believe that knowing is better than guessing" (p. 14).

Professional Norms

In the practice of speech-language pathology and/or audiology an attitude of clinical accountability ensures that practitioners, as a group and as individuals, are responsible and answerable for the services they provide. Accountability implies a process of continuous review and requires the justification of professional activities in terms of the cost, quality, and outcome of care. Douglass (1983) describes the precepts involved in accountability as follows:

1. The welfare of the patient is paramount.
2. A regimen of treatment is followed that, in essence, consists of systematically applied procedures.
3. The ability of a professional, as demonstrated in knowledge and skills, is directly related to the capacity to be helpful to a client.
4. Members of a profession are answerable for their actions on behalf of their clients.
5. The clinical activities of members of a profession must be accounted for or explained in some formal manner. (pp. 107–108)

As speech-language pathologists, we are accountable first and foremost to our clients. According to Douglass, other groups or individuals who hold us accountable include governmental and legal agencies, professional societies, and employers. These groups often define or influence our standards of accountability.

A related primary feature of a professional attitude is a sense of ethical commitment. This commitment reflects a set of internalized values that shape professional behavior whether in the classroom, the lab, or the clinic. It results in a demand for excellence in private and public standards of care and responsibility.

Ethics refers, among other things, to normative principles or rules of conduct that govern acceptable professional practice. Ethics represent a form of professional regulation via individuals' implementation and monitoring of these values. Ethics describe human actions as desirable or undesirable, morally right or wrong, good or bad (Green, 1986). Issues concerning confidentiality of information obtained from and about clients, research with human subjects, informed consent about speech-language pathology services, our professional responsibilities to clients and co-workers, the procurement of fees and financial sponsorship, the use of advertising, and the dispensing of products are examples of ethical considerations (Flower, 1984; Van Hattum & Nikoloff, 1985).

The complete ASHA Code of Ethics is available in the *Membership and Certification Handbook* or in the *Membership Directory* and is reprinted annually in the journal *Asha*. All ASHA members, as well as those individuals who retain the Certificate of Clinical Competence in Speech-Language Pathology and/or Audiology, are bound by its standards. Although not yet ASHA members or certified professionals, students entering the fields of speech-language pathology and audiology should be guided by the principles expressed in the code of ethics.

These ethical principles were not forced upon us by external groups or agencies. The need to create formal ethical standards to regulate professional practice and maintain high-quality clinical service was one of the reasons our association was founded (Paden, 1970). The ASHA Code of Ethics represents our long-held and tested values and the professional attitudes to which we aspire. These principles define us as professionals.

Professional Identity

David Yoder, 1984 ASHA president, commented on the relatively small proportion of school clinicians who are ASHA members and concluded that "we have not marketed well the need for some type of 'professional group membership' to the individual who has graduated from our graduate programs in communication disorders" (p. 37). Membership in ASHA and other state or local groups is not compulsory; yet, in our opinion, the development and preservation of a professional attitude necessitates affiliations of this sort. Professional organizations serve a number of functions and offer many benefits, some of which have already been described (see chapter 1). Perhaps most critical to one's professional posture are the feeling of belonging; the collective sharing of interests, beliefs, and needs; and the sense of collegial commitment and loyalty that membership provides. An organizational structure such as ASHA establishes and preserves our position as a legitimate profession not only to the group members but also to other professional and public groups. The authentication of speech-language pathology and audiology as two areas of professional practice is in actuality an individual matter. That is, each of us represents the group as much or more than the group can represent us. The letters and reports we write, the conversations we hold, and the manner and form of our case management are used as measures of both our personal skills and of the profession as a whole. Individuals who invest the most time and energy in a professional group usually feel that they have gained the most. Professional membership is viewed as a privilege and a responsibility; perhaps it is also an obligation.

Legal Identity

Green (1986) describes licensure as "the process by which a state government agency defines the *scope of practice* within a profession, specifies qualifications for practitioners, and permits individual practitioners to use certain *titles*" (p. 144). For the general public and particularly the communicatively handicapped public, professional licensing provides assurance that an individual has met the minimum standards required by state law to practice a profession. Although licensure does not guarantee quality care, some argue that it protects the consumer better than any other form of regulation (Gross, 1978). For the professionals, these laws establish a legal identity or professional title, contribute to their professional autonomy, recognize their unique qualifications, and thereby establish their right to practice. Legal status may also offer some economic advantages and professional prestige by qualifying its holders to obtain payments from third-party insurers. In addition, licensure demarcates our professional territory and claims a certain portion of the market exclusively for us (Lecomte, 1986). The granting of a license is in some ways pro forma in that ASHA certification standards usually serve as the basis for licensure requirements. Students should become familiar with the licensing law of the state in which they intend to practice because a license is increasingly becoming an admission ticket to professional clinical practice.

Business Acumen

Cooper (1982) in describing his lover's quarrel with the profession of speech-language pathology quoted Chayet, an analyst of the health-care field, who in a paper presented at the 1978 ASHA Directors Conference suggested that our professional doctrine might be "speech-language pathologists and audiologists shall be poor" (cited in Cooper, 1982, p. 932). Less than a decade later a significant number of ASHA members have become increasingly interested in the business aspects of professional practice. Advertising, once prohibited in the ASHA Code of Ethics, is now permissible. The proscription once placed on the dispensing of products such as hearing aids, therapy programs, and assistive devices has been lifted. The private-practice sector of our profession was once repressed but is now gaining substantial support and prestige. Some have argued that our economic survival depends in part on the development of clinical-administration and financial-management skills in our practitioners (Feldman, 1981; Goldman & Levy, 1982). However, human-services professionals have not unanimously supported the image of clinician as businessperson or entrepreneur. Concerns are based in part on the view that all too many businesspersons are "only out to make a buck." After all, as Gerstman (1986) notes, "The objective of business is to seek an advantage (i.e., a profit)" (p. 222). One physician in his mid-sixties remarked:

> The physician going into practice today quickly becomes a businessman. He already knows about health insurance, the ins and outs of third party payments, and the importance of an accountant to tell you how to beat the tax laws. Patients are persons, but they are also fees. (Sarason, 1985, p. 173)

The mention of fees, costs, and budgets may bring either resentment or applause, but these topics cannot be ignored. The health-services system has become an industry. Although our prime focus as clinicians should, of course, be on quality of care, we must recognize the need to value appropriately the services we provide and charge for those services at a fair and equitable rate. Until we do this, we will not be fully accorded our proper professional status.

Personal Qualities

The purpose of this section is not to provide more tips on how to dress for success. We simply wish to reinforce what you already know—you need to conform to certain standards if you want to convey a professional attitude. We understand fully that many regard such standards of personal conduct as dress codes to be degrading and restrictive, and we were very tempted to summarize our feelings about this topic with "Vive la différence!" Nevertheless, most of the established professions maintain remarkably uniform standards for personal appearances. Van Hattum (1985) argued that "if we are to attain our correct position among the professions we must be aware that our appearance and our actions are important." He identified a number of personal qualities observed in the successful speech-language pathologist, including humility and modesty, a healthy and well-groomed appearance, honesty, friendliness, cheerfulness, tactfulness, courteousness, patience, enthusiasm, tolerance, cooperation, dependability, literacy, articulateness, introspectiveness, creativity, and objectivity (pp. 14–23). Neidecker (1987) cites some of these traits and adds those of understanding, resourcefulness, flexibility, adaptability, and a sense of humor. Although these descriptions may sound similar to the virtues of girl scouts, the issues at hand are those of images and impressions. How do you wish to be viewed? This question must be considered in light of the needs of a client group diverse in cultural background, ethnicity, and race; the values and customs of colleagues; the location and climate of the work place; and the strength of institutional traditions.

Blumer (1966) provides a valuable insight on the aims of professionalization and the nature of professional standards.

> Professionalization seeks to clothe a given area with standards of excellence, to establish rules of conduct, to develop a sense of responsibility, to set criteria for recruitment and training, to ensure a measure of protection for members, to establish collective control over the area, and to elevate it to a position of dignity and social standing in the society. (p. xi)

In reality, a professional attitude may be more of a complex and ever-changing goal than an essential feature of the clinical practice of speech-language pathology. We have identified a number of distinctive but related traits and skills that, taken together, may define the ideal type of professional attitude. Students and certified practitioners alike need to examine the attitudes they observe and those they exhibit as professionals.

To professionalism!

■ SUMMARY

In this chapter three attitudes or orientations to clinical practice were identified and described. Our view, as expressed by these attitudes, is that the practitioner must bring to the therapeutic relationship scientific principles as well as the sometimes intangible and often misunderstood qualities of professionalism and compassion. All three attitudes are essential components of high-quality clinical work.

ACTIVITIES

1. Think of a time when you observed a therapy session or other type of clinical interaction involving a clinician you most admire. Identify three outstandingly effective behaviors of this clinician.

2. As a class, develop a composite picture from the behaviors identified for question 1.

3. Categorize these behaviors according to one of the three attitudes (scientific, therapeutic, professional) they reflect.

4. Of the positive behaviors noted, identify those you have demonstrated in your own clinical work.

5. Think of a time when you observed a therapy session or other type of clinical interaction involving a clinician you least admire. Identify three particularly ineffective behaviors of this clinician.

6. As a class, develop a composite picture from the behaviors identified for question 4.

7. Categorize these behaviors according to one of the three attitudes (scientific, therapeutic, professional) they reflect.

8. Of the negative behaviors noted, identify those you have demonstrated in your own clinical work.

9. Read an article published within the past five years that addresses scientific models, methods, or concepts related to a therapy approach you are using, have used, or have seen used.

10. Examine the manual of a published therapy program often used at your clinic. As a class, discuss the adequacy of the information provided by the authors about the scientific basis of this tool.

REFERENCES

Barlow, D., & Hersen, M. (1984). *Single-case experimental designs.* New York: Pergamon.

Bauer, H. (1985). Single-subject research designs in communicative interaction and disorders. *Seminars in Speech and Language, 6*(1), 67–102.

Blumer, H. (1966). Preface. In H. M. Vollmer and D. L. Mills (Eds.), *Professionalization.* Englewood Cliffs, NJ: Prentice-Hall.

Cole, P. (1987). *Asha* interviews Patricia R. Cole. *Asha, 29*(1), 22–26.

Cooper, E. B. (1982). The state of the profession and what to do about it: One lover's quarrel. *Asha, 24*(11), 931–934.

Darley, F. L. (1985). The "heart" of clinical education. *Proceedings of the sixth annual conference on graduate education* (pp. 10–14). St. Louis, MO: Council on Graduate Education.

Douglass, R. (1983, May). Defining and describing clinical accountability. *Seminars in Speech and Language, 4*(2), 107–118.

Eisenstadt, (1972). Weakness in clinical procedures–A parental evaluation. *Asha, 14*(1), 7–9.

Elliot, E. (1984, August). My name is Mrs. Simon. *Ladies Home Journal,* pp. 18, 21, 150.

Feldman, A. S. (1981). The challenge of autonomy: presidential address. *Asha, 23*(12), 941–945.

Flower, R. M. (1984). *Delivery of speech-language pathology services.* Baltimore, MD: Williams & Wilkins.

———. (1985). Asking questions. *Asha, 27*(12), 21–25.

Gerstman, H. L. (1986). Business aspects of management. In R. M. McLauchlin (Ed.), *Speech-language pathology and audiology: issues and management* (pp. 221–265) Orlando, FL: Grune & Stratton.

Goldman, R., & Levy, J. (1982). Economic survival underlines professional public service. *Asha, 24*(2), 103–105.

Green, W. W. (1986). Professional standards and ethics. In R. M. McLauchlin (Ed.), *Speech-language pathology and audiology: Issues and management* (pp. 135–159). Orlando, FL: Grune & Stratton.

Gross, S. J. (1978). The myth of professional licensing. *American Psychologist, 33*(1), 1009–1016.

Hegde, M. (1985). *Treatment procedures in communication disorders.* San Diego, CA: College-Hill Press.

Hildebrand, J. (1957). *Science in the making.* New York: Columbia University Press.

Kamhi, A. (1984). Problem solving in child language disorders: The clinician as clinical scientist. *Language, Speech and Hearing Services in Schools, 15*(4), 226–234.

Kent, R. (1985). Science and the clinician: The practice of science and the science of practice. *Seminars in Speech and Language, 6*(1), 1–12.

Kent, R., & Fair, J. (1985). Clinical research: Who, where, what? *Seminars in Speech and Language, 6*(1), 23–24.

Krupat, E. (1986, November). Physicians and patients: A delicate imbalance. *Psychology Today,* pp. 22, 24–26.

Lecomte, C. (1986). Licensing. In G. S. Tryon (Ed.), *The professional practice of psychology.* Norwood, NJ: Ablex.

McCarthy, P., Culpepper, N. B., & Lucks, L. (1986). Variability in counseling experience and training among ESB-accredited programs. *Asha, 28*(9), 49–52.

McReynolds, L., & Kearns, K. (1982). *Single-subject experimental designs in communicative disorders.* Baltimore, MD: University Park Press.

Moore, W. E. (1970). *The professions: Roles and rules.* New York: Russell Sage Foundation.

Neidecker, E. (1987). *School programs in speech-language pathology: Organization and management.* Englewood Cliffs, NJ: Prentice-Hall.

Prutting, C. (1983). Scientific inquiry and communicative disorders: An emerging pardigm across six decades. In T. Gallagher and C. Prutting (Eds.), *Pragmatic assessment and intervention issues in language* (pp. 247–266). San Diego, CA: College-Hill Press.

Ringel, R. (1972). The clinician and the researcher: An artificial dichotomy. *Asha, 14*(7), 351–353.

Ringel, R., Trachtman, L., & Prutting, C. (1984). The science in human communication sciences. *Asha, 26*(12), 33–36.

Sarason, S. B. (1985). *Caring and compassion in clinical practice.* San Francisco, CA: Jossey-Bass.

Shorter, E. (1985). *Bedside manners.* New York: Simon & Schuster.

Siegel, G., & Ingham, R. (1987). Theory and science in communication disorders. *Journal of Speech and Hearing Disorders, 52*(2), 99–104.

Switzer, E. (1985, June). The failure of America's hospitals. *Ladies Home Journal.*

Van Hattum, R. J. (1985). Introduction. In R. J. Van Hattum (Ed.), *Organization of speech-language services in schools: A manual.* San Diego, CA: College-Hill Press.

West, R. W. (1961). To our new members—*ave et vale. Asha, 3*(1), 6–8.

Yoder, D. E. (1984). President's page, *Asha, 26*(9), 37–38.

CHAPTER FOUR

Clinical Intervention: The Service Spectrum

INTRODUCTION

The following description of speech-language pathology and audiology services appears in the rehabilitation services section of the *Accreditation Manual for Hospitals/87* (JCAH, 1986):

> Speech-language pathology and/or audiology services provide for a continuum of services, including prevention, identification, diagnosis, consultation, and the treatment of patients regarding speech, language, oral and pharyngeal sensorimotor function, hearing, and balance.
>
> Services include, but need not be limited to, the following:
>
> - Screening to identify individuals who require further evaluation to determine the presence or absence of a communicative disorder;
> - Evaluating and diagnosing speech, language, and oral and pharyngeal sensorimotor competencies by a qualified speech-language pathologist, and evaluating and diagnosing auditory and vestibular competencies by a qualified audiologist using instrumentation such as audiometers, electroacoustic immittance equipment, evoked potential response equipment, and electronystagmographic equipment;
> - Planning, directing, and conducting habilitative, rehabilitative, and counseling programs to treat disorders of verbal and written language, voice, articulation, fluency, interactive communication, mastication, deglutition,

auditory and/or visual processing and memory, and cognition/communication; and assisted, and/or augmentative communication treatment and devices; and

- Planning, directing, and conducting aural habilitation and rehabilitation programs by the audiologist.

Such programs may include, but need not be limited to:

- The selection of and orientation to hearing aids and assistive listening devices;
- Counseling, guidance, and auditory training;
- Speech reading; and
- Language habilitation.

The professional develops discharge plans and strives to ensure the patient's understanding of his communication abilities and prognosis.

Speech-language and/or audiology services are monitored to determine the effectiveness of actions taken to improve patients' communication skills. (pp. 238–239)

The term *continuum* used to describe the many clinical services provided by speech-language pathologists and audiologists captures the ongoing nature of these services but also suggests that they follow a natural order. We propose, instead, that these services constitute a spectrum involving a series of dynamic and related processes. Although services may be organized separately and sequentially for purposes of billing, student training, documenting attendance, or writing chapters like this one, in reality these services are inseparable. At any given moment a service may appear anywhere along the spectrum. At times, services may be indistinguishable or even reciprocal. For example, tradition and practice dictate that effective treatment be based on accurate assessment. Yet, a diagnosis is at best only an approximation of an individual's status based on historical data and current performance. In treatment, diagnosis is ongoing and evolves over time. Decisions may be refined or reversed following continued observations of a person's responses and learning preferences. Further, the evaluation itself is therapeutic in that the client may "feel better" and more relaxed or hopeful because a problem was confronted, confirmed, or shared and because help was offered (Meitus, 1983). In reference to evaluation and therapy, Boone (1971) stresses an integral relationship and describes them as overlapping extensively. Over the past decade a number of writers have begun to challenge the temporal and conceptual dichotomy of these activities (Lord, Larson, & McKinley, 1987; Muma, 1978; Rees, 1978; Shultz, 1972). In this sense, assessment and treatment are reciprocal processes that have longitudinal and cross-sectional dimensions. Similar cases may be made about most of our clinical services.

We have chosen to categorize the key services along the spectrum as *prevention, assessment, therapy, discharge planning,* and *consultation.* Each discussion begins with a general definition of the service. Next we identify the objectives or purposes to which such clinical services are directed. We then consider the basic strategies or approaches common to each type of service. Strategies are principles that address what is to be accomplished but do not specify the procedures or methods of implementation. Finally, we describe the format of each service. By format we refer to the form, style, arrangement, or general design of the service. We make such distinctions to help clarify the concepts and contexts of clinical practices.

PREVENTION

Definition

Prevention is an established concept in medicine and public health, but it has only recently gained recognition as a serious clinical endeavor. Although the literature on prevention of communication disorders is not extensive, it offers a reasonable basis for including prevention as an appropriate and desirable form of professional service.

In 1982 the ASHA Committee on the Prevention of Speech, Language, and Hearing Problems addressed the trend in prevention practices with the following statement: "In a general sense, prevention of communicative disorders is the elimination of those causes which interfere with the normal acquisition and development of communication skills" (p. 425). To recognize the frequent progression in seriousness and degree of disability of communication problems from onset to advanced stages, the committee differentiated between primary, secondary, and tertiary phases of prevention. The primary phase describes intervention with individuals or a targeted population prior to the manifestation of clinical signs of communication difficulties but for which there is statistical support that an inclination toward such problems exists.

The secondary phase pertains to intervention through early detection of emerging clinical symptoms. Tertiary prevention refers to intervention or rehabilitation that forestalls or obviates residual effects or future advancement of the identified problem. Accepted definitions and accompanying examples as taken from the committee report follow:

1. Primary Prevention is the elimination or inhibition of the onset and development of a communicative disorder by altering susceptibility or reducing exposure for susceptible individuals. EXAMPLES: Cigarette smoking is eliminated to prevent future laryngeal and breathing anomalies.
2. Secondary Prevention is the early detection and treatment of communicative disorders. Early detection may lead to elimination of the disorder or the retardation of the disorder's progress, thereby preventing further complications. One of the major practices of secondary prevention is mass screening of persons without symptoms. EXAMPLE: The institution of a school auditory screening program which systematically tests the hearing of all children on a periodic basis and after certain illnesses, such as infectious diseases of the ear.
3. Tertiary Prevention is the reduction of a disability by attempting to restore effective functioning. The major approach is rehabilitation of the disabled individual who has realized some residual problems as a result of the disorder. EXAMPLE: The institution of a program of rehabilitation for a dysphasic patient as soon as possible after the onset of the neuropathology in order to prevent more serious communicative and behavioral problems. (1982, pp. 425, 431)

Objectives

In a general sense, prevention intervention is undertaken by speech-language pathologists to reduce the incidence, or number of new cases, of communication disorders introduced into the existing population over a specified time period (Marge, 1984; ASHA Committee on the Prevention of Speech, Language, and Hearing Problems, 1984). In *Heal Thy People: The Surgeon General's Report on Health Promotion and Disease Prevention* (1979), a germinal paper, goals to be achieved by 1990 were identified. An analysis of these goals by a task force composed of government-agency representatives resulted in the development of 226 national prevention objectives and 12 health-status goals. In a 1984 interview, J. M. McGinnis, then assistant secretary for health and director of the Office of Disease Prevention and Health Promotion in the U.S. Department of Health and Human Services, identified attainment of the 1990 goals as the top prevention priority of the Public Health Service agencies (Staff, 1984). The three prevention activities identified as essential for attainment of the overall goals were (1) health promotion services, (2) health protection services, and (3) individual preventive health services.

Strategies

Marge (1984) examined the concept of prevention relating to clinical practices and presented 13 strategies for prevention intervention with many disabilities, including communicative disorders. These preventive steps as proposed by Marge involve the following:

1. Immunization against infectious diseases such as diphtheria, tetanus, pertussis, rubella, polio, measles, and mumps, some of which are directly linked to speech, language, and hearing disorders
2. Genetic counseling to decrease the number of cases of communication problems linked with certain genetic diseases
3. Prenatal care to maintain the proper intrauterine environment for the delivery of a neurologically intact infant
4. Mass screening and early detection to identify individuals with subtle signs of a disease or disability
5. Early intervention programs to suppress the effects of a known or suspected disorder
6. Family planning to reduce the numbers of unplanned pregnancies
7. Proper medical care of the population at large to monitor health status and again for the purpose of early identification of problems
8. Public education to inform the community about prevention strategies and promote their use

9. Education programs for children and youth to equip youngsters with information about health care, specifically as it relates to communication disorders
10. Environmental quality control to protect the population from the hazards that result from the abuse or misuse of our natural resources
11. Quality-of-life programs to offer support and assistance to individuals entering into or involved in stressful situations or experiences
12. Governmental action to oversee the implementation of prevention programs
13. Reduction of poverty to alleviate the health problems associated with indigence

Examples of prevention activities specific to speech-language pathology and audiology include early identification of and intervention with speech-language problems, participation in antismoking campaigns and noise-pollution programs, the implementation of a vocal abuse reduction program, the development of industrial hearing conservation programs, and the use of support groups with families of individuals who have communication problems. Shadden (1987) described a precrisis intervention model used with the elderly who are at risk for stroke-related communication problems. This novel form of preventive training seeks to reduce the impact of the personal trauma felt by the individual who suffers a stroke and his or her family members and peers. Marge (1981, 1984) provides information about how to plan and implement prevention intervention. The ASHA Committee on the Prevention of Speech, Language, and Hearing Problems compiled a sample list of prevention materials, and it appears in the August 1984 issue of *Asha*.

Format

The format of prevention intervention differs from that of conventional treatment plans and diagnostic evaluation because prevention measures are not designed typically for a particular individual but rather for a community or population. Further, and as pointed out in the 1986 *Special Needs Report* of the Children's Hospital Medical Center of Akron (1986), because prevention approaches seek to prevent primary impairments from contributing to secondary handicaps, they are quite different from remediation programs, which attempt to correct everything that is not right in a child (p. 1). In addition, although prevention approaches are the responsibility of speech-language pathologists and audiologists, they may be initiated by physicians, other health-care providers, or interested members of the community. Weiss and Lillywhite, in their 1981 book entitled *Communicative Disorders: Prevention and Early Intervention,"* point out the need for increased understanding of the developmental processes involved in communication, greater attention to preventive approaches, and early detection and treatment of communicative disorders. This need is still apparent.

ASSESSMENT

Definition

Simply stated, the assessment of communication is a complex process that consists of properly posing and effectively resolving questions. These questions relate to the nature of an individual's behavior and focus on abilities and disabilities. Assessment is a central service of the profession of speech-language pathology and audiology. To us it represents (1) the determination of whether a problem exists; (2) an interpretation of what an individual can or cannot, or perhaps will or will not, do; and (3) a description of how certain behaviors differ from normal, the frequency and degree of difference, and how they are distinguished from other problems. As indicated earlier, assessment represents an ongoing process. Questions lead to answers, but often answers generate new questions. This definition and the discussion that follows apply only to the assessment of individuals, not to programs or settings. In this context, we use the term *assessment* interchangeably with *evaluation*, although this is not consistently done by writers in speech-language pathology.

Objectives

In order to maximize the benefits of the assessment process, we must carefully consider our reasons for utilizing particular diagnostic formats or strategies.

1. Is a problem suspected?

The first goal of assessment is to determine if a speech and/or language problem is suspected; that is, to decide whether an individual's communication pattern needs further study. This step of the assessment process, known as *screening*, typically involves short-term examination of a general population or subgroups in which the prevalence of communication problems is greatest, using quick but discriminating measures. Although the screening process is not generally considered an assessment goal, it satisfies this function for us.

2. Does a speech and/or language problem exist?
3. What are the individual's strengths and weaknesses?

After signs of a speech and/or language problem are identified, the clinician seeks to confirm and describe in detail the characteristics of the individual in terms of strengths and weaknesses. Nation and Aram (1984) suggest three perspectives to be used in the description of an individual's speech and/or language behavior; (1) as a variation, that is, speech and/or language differs from normal expectations but is not aberrant; (2) as a disorder, that is, the speech and/or language behaviors are neither acceptable nor appropriate according to normative criteria; and (3) as a speech and language problem in terms of the severity, or the degree to which the disorder presents a handicap for the client or the client's family.

4. What is causing or contributing to the speech and/or language problem?

Through assessment the practitioner attempts to specify the conditions that cause, contribute to, and/or maintain the problem behaviors. Related to the identification of causative links is the desire to classify a communication problem according to a disorder category or by pathology. Meitus (1983) states that "as a general rule, causes of speech and language disorders should be determined" (p. 24). Because speech is so terrifically complicated, however, neurologic, organic, structural, motivational, social, and educational factors must be considered. Because specific treatments are rarely associated with causal factors of communication problems and etiologies cannot be determined with reasonable degrees of certainty, Rees (1978) discourages the overuse of etiologic labels.

5. Would speech and/or language therapy be useful?
6. What are the specific recommendations for treatment?

Assessment is often conducted in an effort to formulate a treatment plan or assist in program placement decisions. Flower (1984) advises that evaluation should

> lead to at least provisional conclusions about the next steps to be taken toward amelioration of the disorder. These steps may involve seeking the help of other professionals for the treatment of physiologic, psychologic, or social impediments to communication. They may involve the development of a program to help the client acquire improved communication. They may entail planning services that seek to lessen the handicaps that attend irremediable disorders. (p. 9)

Through assessment we often determine whether treatment should be attempted and how, where, and when. Assessment results form the basis of the therapy plan, within which assessment continues as the original presenting problem changes in form and frequency.

7. What is the individual's potential for change?

An important objective of an assessment is to offer professional opinions about the likelihood of further intervention improving communication patterns. Prognostic statements are established in accordance with diagnostic findings and often include information about the length of treatment anticipated. Meitus (1983) explains the use of prognoses in the following manner:

> First, they provide patients and families with statements of expectations regarding communication improvement. Second, they force the clinician into a position of accountability. What is recommended for a patient reflects our clinical predictions. Not all patients will profit from speech-language therapy. It is likely that some patients will improve without intervention. By comparing outcomes with predictions, clinicians can determine both the accuracy of their diagnoses and the appropriateness of their recommendations. (p. 27)

A somewhat different view is offered by Rees (1978), who questioned the legitimacy of assessing the outcome of remediation as part of the initial evaluation.

8. What is the individual's pretreatment status?

Another reason for conducting evaluations is to establish a performance baseline against which to measure change in behavior and to monitor the extent of progress through the course of intervention.

Strategies

Strategies are plans of action for or approaches to accumulating data needed to answer the questions that arise during the assessment process. Assessment information is collected from several sources—some current, others historical—including observations, tests, interviews and reports, and diagnostic treatment.

Observations

Observation is an extremely valuable and crucial assessment strategy. It provides a mechanism for identifying and analyzing an individual's behavior and thus gaining a fuller understanding of his or her performance. Emerick and Haynes (1986) state that "a diagnostic session begins with observation and must ultimately return to observation for validation of the measures obtained" (p. 18). Based on earlier research, they recommend a sequence of five steps in diagnostic observation: focus, depth, description, interpretation, and implications.

Focus is defined as a form of systematic observation in which the observer identifies the specific behaviors observed and counts or otherwise quantifies the frequency, duration, and magnitude with which these behaviors occur. Focus, then, serves to enhance objectivity and reduce perceptual bias.

The *depth* of the observation refers to both the amount of time and the number and variety of settings in which the observation is conducted. Emerick and Haynes (1986) stress the importance of noting the consistency or variability of behaviors and personal interactions across situations and with different participants to validate the accuracy of observation.

Description means the translation of behavioral observations or clinical events. To be effective, descriptions must be highly accurate, specific, explicit, objective, and complete. They must be free from judgment and classification.

Interpretation requires the analysis and evaluation of behaviors previously identified and described. These judgments play a critical role in assessment. As Salvia and Ysseldyke (1978) note, "Judgments represent both the best and the worst of assessment data. Judgments made by conscientious, capable and objective individuals can be an invaluable aid in the assessment process. Inaccurate, biased, subjective judgments can be misleading at best and harmful at worst" (pp. 9–10).

In the final step of observation the observer suggests the meaning or *implications* of the observed behaviors. These inferences often lead to conclusions about etiology and treatment plans.

Nation and Aram (1984) assert that "every activity that occurs in the diagnosis serves as a source of data to be observed; no source of information should go unobserved or be wasted" (p. 158). The importance of this statement cannot be overemphasized.

Tests

A common strategy in assessment is the use of commercially available tests. Tests offer the advantages of being convenient, available, and standardized, and in some cases they include normative data. Tests are especially useful because they allow questions or tasks to be presented in a predetermined and consistent manner to each person tested (Salvia & Ysseldyke, 1978). There are some skill areas or behaviors for which commercially prepared or norm-referenced measures are scarce. For the most part, however, there is an abundance of assessment tools or tests available. The diagnostician must select those believed to be most appropriate and useful for a particular individual, based in part on the assessment questions to be considered. The tests themselves vary in their specific focus (e.g., tests of articulation, language, comprehension, or expression), type (e.g., screening, predictive, diagnostic), adequacy (e.g., reliability and validity), originality, ease of administration, and versatility.

Salvia and Ysseldyke (1978) propose that tests yield both quantitative and qualitative information. The quantitative data take the form of actual scores or derived scores, whereas the qualitative information provides a description of test behavior and of how scores were obtained.

Interviews/Reports

Assessment interviews are conducted to share information with and gather information about the client. Historically, interviews with the client as informant have been considered basic to assessment. Interviews may vary in format, content, information obtained from the client, and the method or process through which this information is obtained. Conventionally, however, interviews are performed to establish rapport, clarify the purpose of the assessment, identify the problem or complaint from the client's perspective, obtain historical data, and offer support. Case-history questionnaires completed by the client or a family member serve as a supplement to or a springboard for the diagnostic interview.

Speech-language pathologists may obtain assessment information from such individuals as family members, teachers, psychologists, and physicians, as well as through direct statements made by the client. The professional and personal opinions offered by these individuals can play a significant part in the assessment process. Other professionals may refer an individual to the speech-language pathologist for evaluation or may be contacted by us to enhance or confirm our findings. The reasons for making a referral affect the design of an assessment session, the development of our clinical hypotheses, and ultimately the selection of assessment tools. Accounts by clients or family members can provide us with information about previous evaluations, developmental background, and medical history. Reporters have their own special perspectives based in part on their training, relationships with the client, and unwittingly, on their own background. The clinician must incorporate these various viewpoints with his or her own observation and test data to arrive at a clinical decision.

Diagnostic Treatment

Baxter, Cohen, and Ylvisaker (1985) use the term *diagnostic treatment* to refer to the systematic exploration of factors that may influence learning and performance. In diagnostic treatment the clinician introduces one or several therapy methods and evaluates the client's responses. The clinician may also identify specific aspects of the client's learning style and analyze patterns and changes following the presentation of varying conditions. For example, some of the factors that must be considered with a traumatically head-injured child include the learning environment; the endurance, persistence, and initiative of the client; the explicitness of rules and instructions; and the types of reinforcement (p. 251).

Format

By definition, a format is a general plan for the organization and arrangement of something. There is no single format for assessment that is accepted or practiced by all speech-language pathologists. Rather, assessment varies in structure, such as formal versus informal; form, such as direct versus indirect; and for several other reasons, such as place of employment, need for referral, and the primary purpose of the assessment.

Structure

Assessment may be arranged formally or informally. Formal assessment often connotes the use of commercially prepared tests. These tools are formal in the sense that directions, administration, and scoring are consistent or standardized across examiners and clients, and the technical features of the test (reliability, validity, and norms) are reported. The examiner must adhere strictly to the information in the test manual to interpret results precisely. A formal structure is commonly used when the primary objective of an evaluation is screening.

Informal assessment includes interviews, structured observation, and clinician-made tests. These procedures are casual and subjective only in that they do not offer the rigorous format of standardized tests and that they can be adapted to the needs, moods, and strengths of the clients. In regard to informal observations, Nation and Aram (1984), who prefer the term *guided observations*, offer the following excellent discussion:

At times the stimuli presented are rigorously controlled; at other times, they are controlled only in a general sense. For example, when a patient is asked to sit down, stand up, or hop, skip, and jump, the diagnostician has controlled his stimuli to specify a response. He may want to observe the patient's motor abilities and or his ability to follow directions. If the plan is to obtain as much spontaneous speech as naturalistically as possible, the diagnostician's stimulus specification may be more general; that is, the diagnostician bases his conversational stimuli on the patient's spontaneous conversation. But the diagnostician's observation of this conversation may be highly planned and structured to obtain specific speech and language data. (p. 158)

Informal assessment is of particular merit when the objective of assessment is to describe the speech and language behaviors.

Form

When observations, tests, and interviews are conducted by the diagnostician, a direct form of assessment occurs. In contrast, an indirect form of assessment exists when information is collected from another person (e.g., parents, guardians, teachers, and various health professionals) or through analysis of the educational system or home environment. Assessment of the home environment involves an examination not only of peer and family characteristics but of wide-ranging variables. For example, Lord, Larson, and McKinley (1987) considered four major areas of assessment in the educational system of an adolescent. These include the structure or flexibility of the system, the teacher's language, teachers' and administrators' attitudes toward students with communication disorders, and curriculum variables (p. 129).

By using interviews, observations, checklists, attitude scales, rating scales, curriculum-analysis measures, and so forth, the assessor can gain valuable insight about the nature, cause, and prognosis of the problem. Diagnosticians may need or wish to rely on others to obtain information about behaviors that occur infrequently or only within particular environments or with certain individuals.

Assessment Variables

A number of factors may influence the assessment format, including the major goal(s) of assessment, the work setting, characteristics of the client, and the reason for referral. Obviously, certain objectives lend themselves more to one form or structure of assessment than another. In particular, the effects of such factors as the evaluation site, or employment settings, and/or the reason for the evaluation referral can be demonstrated in terms of length, frequency, and focus of assessment. According to Nation and Aram (1984),

Various amounts of time are allotted to the diagnostic process in different settings. Time, therefore, becomes an important practical consideration in using the steps of the method. In one setting the entire process may be restricted in an hour's duration; in others, several hours or repeated sessions may be permitted. (p. 63)

The age, primary disorder, disposition, physical capabilities, and cultural background of the client are examples of client characteristics that may influence—if not dictate—assessment practices. Some clients may be able to tolerate only brief, frequent diagnostic sessions. Others may require adaptations of test materials because of their physical and/or motor limitations or their linguistic and/or cultural differences.

The reason for referral should also affect the format of assessment. Nation and Aram (1984) point out, some referrals are made for the purpose of screening large groups of individuals, whereas others request information about the efficacy of treatment, the likely causes of the problem, or a plan to be implemented in another context. These examples represent only several of the many ways in which assessment formats vary and reasons that they do.

THERAPY

Definition

What exactly is *therapy*? Therapy can be viewed as often rewarding, sometimes frustrating, frequently exciting, and occasionally sobering. It is an act of compassion and a form of objective conduct, a dynamic process and a structured task, an offer of assistance and a lesson in independence, an adventure and a business, an art and a science. In plain terms, therapy means "to serve." Holland (1983) provides a delightful characterization of the therapy process, which we will paraphrase: it is rolling up your sleeves and doing whatever your principles, your training, your skills, your sensitivity, and finally, your patients themselves tell you needs to be done to make the communicative world a little more natural for them (p. 13).

Flower (1984) defines therapy as comprising all activities that are carried out in an effort to modify communicative behaviors. He classifies these activities according to three categories that represent the primary goal of therapy.

Objectives

According to Flower (1984), therapy activities can be grouped into three broad and overlapping goal categories, which include the following:

1. Activities aimed at the mastery of specific components of normal communication processes
2. Activities aimed at the achievement of compensation for irremediable impairments
3. Activities aimed at changing attitudinal barriers to better communication (pp. 9–10)

The first goal reflects those actions taken to improve one or more of the specific aspects (e.g., phonologic, semantic, syntactic, pragmatic), more general features (e.g., voice, fluency, rate), and modalities (e.g., reading, writing, speaking) of communication. As an illustration, therapy might focus on the specific behaviors of producing a particular sound, or more broadly on improving overall intelligibility, or on comprehending written materials. The second goal involves the development of new strategies or alternatives to normal communication processes in the face of a permanent or long-term problem. Examples include mechanical devices such as hearing aids for the deaf or hearing impaired, communication boards for the nonspeaking population, and artificial larynxes and other speech appliances for the laryngectomized. Compensatory and/or instructional techniques also fall within this category and include the following examples: requests that a speaker repeat or slow down a message to facilitate language processing, written cues or gestures to facilitate word retrieval, log books to compensate for impaired memory, speech reading to compensate for a hearing handicap, sign language to provide a means of communication for the deaf, and Amerind as a communication mode for clients with apraxia of speech (see Flower, 1984, and Szekeres, Ylvisaker, and Holland, 1985, among others, for additional examples). The third goal refers to efforts made by the clinician to modify the client's self-defeating behaviors and explore suitable ways to modify performance. Flower cites two examples related to this goal: (1) helping an aphasic overcome the fear of making speech errors, as manifested in overmonitoring of communication or reluctance to communicate, and (2) helping the hearing-impaired individual who is too embarrassed to wear a hearing aid accept both the disability and the device that will ease it. This goal, then, enables the client to use his or her skills or compensatory mechanisms to change behavior.

We would add two other goals of therapy: the first is directed toward helping the client and his or her family accept, adjust to, cope with, or control those stresses related to or resulting from a communication problem or a new communication style. The integral role of counseling in the therapy process has been repeatedly described in the literature and will be discussed further in the next section of this chapter on therapy strategies. A final goal category represents those activities aimed at changing or manipulating the environment in which the individual communicates. Within the classroom, the work setting, or the place of residence, the clinician may decrease or eliminate factors that perpetuate or confound a problem. The clinician may also increase appropriate reinforcement, improve the individual's "access to learning" (Ripich & Spinelli, 1985), and, where appropriate, increase or decrease acceptance of the problem.

Strategies

As clinicians, we quickly discover that diversity rather than uniformity reflects the state of the art in speech and language therapy. Nevertheless, we have strived in our discussion to describe comprehensive approaches or broad strategies that are still in general use, are not disorder or age specific, and are the basis for a variety of specific clinical activities. We will discuss several clinical strategies, including the operant approaches, perceptual and cognitive process orientations,

counseling, compensatory training, social modeling, and ethnographic intervention. These approaches are not mutually exclusive, nor are they the only clinical
strategies in use. They are, however, representative of those that have
predominated.

Operant Strategies

The clinical applications of behaviorist, or programmed-operant, models are quite
prevalent. Briefly, operant behavior is behavior emitted voluntarily by the client
that produces a consequence in his or her environment. The individual's perception of these consequences will influence the frequency of his or her behaviors.
That is, if the person views the consequence as pleasant, the behavior or response
is reinforced and thus learned and is likely to recur. Conversely, if the person
views the consequence as unpleasant, the behavior tends not to be repeated.
Operant conditioning, sometimes referred to as instrumental conditioning, is a
highly controlled procedure in which environmental variables or stimuli are
manipulated so as to increase, decrease, or maintain designated behaviors.

The three major steps in a programmed-operant model include (1) obtaining
baseline measures of behavior prior to treatment; (2) applying conditioning
procedures to change the behavior or establish a new behavior; and (3) transferring, or "carrying over," of the newly learned behavior from controlled to more
natural situations (LaPointe, 1985). Many examples exist of clinical strategies that
reflect operant theory. Some clinicians apply specific learning principles—such as
positive reinforcement, negative reinforcement, modeling, shaping, fading, pun-
ishment, extinction, stimulus control, and contingency management—more often
than others. The range of our use of these strategies extends from the verbal
praise provided after successful articulation of a particular sound or word choice
to the administration of a commercially available programmed-operant method.

Two behavioral techniques used commonly in the clinical situation are
contingency management and *behavioral modeling*. Contingency management refers
to the organization of a session so that the client knows that a reward is dependent
on the demonstration of a desired behavior or completion of a certain task. The
reward or reinforcement must, of course, be of sufficient value that it motivates
the client to perform. Behavioral modeling involves the use of a reward to
encourage immediate imitation of a specific behavior or a designated model (see
Gearheart, 1973). This represents a very common form of instruction, although
its implementation is not always systematic.

Although clinical approaches based on operant theory were at their peak in
the sixties and seventies, they are still popular today. Shames and Egolf (1976)
offer this interesting observation:

> We have come to realize that operant strategies really introduce no new content to
> our work, but rather dispose us toward more precise observation and definition,
> toward greater consistency in our behavior as clinicians, and toward developing
> more objective ways of evaluating the processes and results of therapy. (p. 20)

For extensive discussions of the operant approach and examples of its application in speech-language pathology, readers are referred to Alberto and Troutman (1986), Fey (1986), Hegde (1985), Shames and Egolf (1976), and Winokur (1976).

Social Modeling

Social learning theory contends that most human behavior is acquired through observation of modeled events. Whereas behavioral modeling assumes the use of reinforcement, social modeling emphasizes the ways in which social and personal factors influence an individual's attention and motivation and ultimately his or her ability to learn. Fey (1986), discussing language intervention with children, outlined five steps typically followed in approaches based on social learning theory: (1) select a model with whom the client closely identifies, such as a parent or peer; (2) have the model produce numerous examples of the target behavior; (3) reward the model for correct performance; (4) after the presentation of several uninterrupted models, encourage the client to "talk just like the model"; and (5) reinforce the client for correct performance (p. 13).

Fey asserts that a fundamental difference between the behavioral and social learning approaches is that the immediate imitation of each modeled stimulus required by the first is not a necessary component of the second. In fact, social learning theorists view immediate imitation as a potential interference with the client's internal processing of new information.

We borrow this clinical example from Fey (1986):

> In a naturalistic intervention context, when an appropriate situation for language usage by the child arises, a behaviorist must feel compelled to prompt the child to produce a complete target response. In contrast, a social learning theorist may feel content to (1) provide models of the target, some of which are overtly reinforced; (2) see that other children produce models of the target response under similar circumstances; and (3) model the correct response, following the child's incorrect attempts. It is not essential for the child to produce a response to assume that learning is taking place. All that is necessary is that the environmental (social and physical) conditions be modified such that the child is highly motivated to pay attention to these models and the objects, states, events, and relations to which they refer. The clinician's role is changed from one of the elicitor and reinforcer of specific responses to one of modeler and motivator of language usage. (p. 14)

Readers seeking additional information about social learning theory are referred to Fey (1986), Bandura (1977), and Courtright and Courtright (1976).

Perceptual and Cognitive Process Approaches

Holland (1983) used the term *process approaches* to describe treatment strategies that attempt to modify the processes underlying language. We have adopted this term because it is broad enough to include cognitive, sensory, and perceptual orientations. In discussing language intervention in adults, Holland identified four processes that have been the focus of therapy in this context: (1) enrichment of auditory and visual perceptions, (2) the reorganization and reintegration of cortical functions (e.g., the use of movement to initiate speech-related activities), (3) the enhancement of verbal memory, and (4) the engagement of the right hemisphere (pp. 5–7). Examples of clinical approaches that reflect this rationale include visual-imagery or visual-sequencing training to improve memory, melodic intonation therapy for treating apraxia of speech, and auditory training in dealing with language learning disabilities.

Ethnographic, Sociolinguistic, or Naturalistic Approaches

Ethnography refers to methods of analyzing events and persons that enable us to determine the underlying rules operative for the participants in a particular culture (e.g., classroom, social group) (Ripich & Spinelli, 1985). That is, through ethnographic or sociolinguistic methodologies, we are able to understand better how an individual with a communication problem interacts with others in an instructional and/or social setting. In the case of a child, participants in therapy may include the child, teacher, peers, and clinician. An intervention plan for an adult may involve a spouse, other family member, or co-worker. Ethnographic approaches are based on the assumption that it is essential to examine events in their natural environments and to study the nature or the process of the interaction, rather than the result (Ripich & Spinelli, 1985; Wilson, 1977). Naturalistic observations typically involve audio and/or video recordings in combination with a participant's observational notes (Weitz, 1985). Wilkinson, Clevenger, and Dollaghan (1981) point out that the ethnographer describes not only verbal but also nonverbal performance.

Increasing interest in pragmatic and discourse goals and in alternate models of service delivery, such as home health care or classroom-based therapy, has contributed to increased use of ethnographic approaches. Examples of specific therapy techniques related to ethnographic theory include the modification of the directions used by a teacher to instruct the child in the classroom; the utilization of a spouse or sibling to prompt appropriate communication behavior; and the manipulation of the content, rate, or amount of parental language to increase fluent speech. Spinelli and Ripich (1983) provide an intervention approach designed to modify both a teacher's instructional messages and a language-disordered child's responses to these instructions.

Milieu or environmental therapy as described by Haarbauer-Krupa, Moser, Smith, Sullivan, and Szekeres (1985) captures in many ways the essence of an ethnographic approach. According to these authors, milieu therapy considers the complexity, rate, and duration of the stimuli in the rehabilitation setting or home environment; the appropriateness of activities in which the client is expected to participate; the family and staff input and response to the client's communication attempts; and daily routines and events in which the client engages. Additional information about ethnograhic treatment approaches may be found in Cherry (1978), Cook-Gumperz and Gumperz (1982), Lund and Duchan (1983), Mehan (1982), and Ripich and Spinelli (1985).

Compensatory Training

Unfortunately, not all communication impairments can be corrected. Some clients may never grow out of their problems but instead adapt to their problems by using certain compensatory devices, examples of which were given earlier. Haarbauer-Krupa, Henry, Szekeres, and Ylvisaker (1985) offer a compensatory training paradigm consisting of three phases. In phase one, general strategic thinking, clients are made aware of their deficits and the implications of these and are taught the value of using compensatory strategies. The second phase, teaching the strategy, involves providing the clients with tasks for monitoring their use of compensatory strategies, having the clinician or a peer model the steps in a strategy, and explaining clearly the purpose and use of the strategy to clients. The final phase of this plan focuses on the generalization and maintenance of a strategy beyond the training context (pp. 318–319). This focus of intervention is relatively new but has been used with head-injured and language learning disabled children.

Nonspeech intervention illustrates another type of compensatory training. Individuals unable to talk because of severe cognitive, motor, or emotional difficulties use communication devices—some electronically simple, others technologically sophisticated—to reveal their thoughts and to interact with others. Clients may also receive assistance in augmenting their speech or compensating for irreversible disorders through the use of writing, typing, drawing, gesturing, pantomiming, or signing (Jaffe, Mastrilli, Molitor, & Valko, 1985). There is a growing body of literature on the use of augmentative or alternative methods of communication (e.g., Blackstone, 1986; Carlson, 1981; Goldman & Dahle, 1985; Grossfield & Grossfield, 1986; Katz, 1986; Meyers, 1984; Minifie, 1984; Sanders, J. 1986; Schwarz, 1984; Shane & Sauer, 1986; and Silverman, 1987).

Counseling

Counseling refers to those services provided to clients or their families to ease the emotional stress or interpersonal crises arising from, contributing to, or somehow associated with primary communication problems. Counseling can be directed toward helping the client or family adjust to the sudden onset or discovery of a communication problem (as in the case of aphasia, head injury, hearing loss, or birth defects such as cleft palate), to accept the permanence of a speech or language handicap, to resolve conflicts that may cause or contribute to communication difficulties, and to support therapy goals. Flower (1984) points out that counseling may also enable clients to recognize and gain assistance for other areas of functioning in which they need help, for example, with medical, psychiatric, and vocational difficulties. Preparation of prospective clients for therapy may also be viewed as one part of the counseling process. The speech-language pathologist or audiologist may provide the counseling or call upon another specialist to assist. In a sense, all therapy should involve counseling as epitomized by our continuous attempts to understand clients and to increase

clients' self-understanding. McWilliams (1976), describing aspects of parent counseling, contends that "every professional person who interacts with parents and
children becomes a counselor. The role may vary from parent to parent; and the
methodology may be, indeed should be, based upon the clinician's assessment
of the parents' requirements at a particular time" (p. 27). A common goal of
counseling is to provide the client with a supportive relationship in which he or
she will be willing to take chances, to expose vulnerabilities, and to make positive
changes.

Counseling approaches vary from informal dialogues to formal therapy and
group sessions and/or educational programs. Services may include the provision
of general information about the disorder and its treatment, the offer of specific
insights about the client's particular communication behaviors, or direct confrontation of psychological problems (Shadden, 1987, p. 66). Several counseling
techniques have emerged from many different schools of therapy. Some of these
approaches include confrontation, desensitization, reinforcement, relaxation therapy, role playing, and bibliotherapy. Differences in counseling techniques are
beyond the scope of this chapter; however, the reader can review current
counseling considerations in communication disorders in the following sources:
Bloom, Johnson, Bitler, and Christman (1986); McFarlane, Fujiki, and Brinton
(1984); and Webster (1977).

In summary, a number of prominent theoretical models have been presented
which differ to some extent in their orientations and methods and offer clinicians
a variety of service options. Attempts to modify an individual's communication
may involve changes in any one or a combination of the following:

1. The client's skills (Intervention strategies might include, for example,
   operant approaches, compensatory training, or social modeling.);
2. The processes that are said to underlie these skills (with intervention
   through perceptual and cognitive process orientations);
3. The environment or factors external to the client (with intervention
   through compensatory training, ethnographic intervention, and
   counseling);
4. The emotional and social support systems (with intervention through
   counseling).

The clinician's choice of strategies must take into account the client's ability
to change. In this regard, a number of factors must be considered, including the
client's age, strengths and weaknesses, motivation, degree of impairment, and
available resources. These factors relate not only to this section on therapy
strategies but also to the various therapy formats addressed in the next section of
this chapter.

Format

In an attempt to satisfy the different needs of individuals with communication
problems clinicians have created a number of varied therapy formats. These

formats will be distinguished according to number (individual versus group), form (direct versus indirect), and setting (classroom, home, or clinic).

Number

Individual therapy involves one speech-language pathologist working with one client. Many advocate this one-client-to-one-clinician format, especially for young or severely handicapped children, because each client demonstrates individual strengths and weaknesses (Hughes, 1985). Group therapy, as might be expected, refers to a speech-language pathologist working with more than one client in a particular session. Group therapy, sometimes criticized as inefficient, has recently been touted as more efficient for both client and clinician and more effective for the client than individual therapy (McCormick & Schiefelbusch, 1984). It has also been suggested that group therapy may facilitate generalization (Hughes, 1985; Oliver & Scott, 1981). Leith (1984) presented a humorous portrayal of group models, which he distinguishes as "mob therapy, therapy in groups and group therapy" (p. 123). According to Leith, group therapy implies an interaction between the members of the group. It also implies that the members of the group are directly involved in the therapeutic process, both in terms of receiving therapy and providing therapy (p. 124).

In creating a group, one must consider the characteristics, skills, and background of its members. Factors such as familiarity with or relation to the client; the type, severity, and degree of the disorder, and intellectual abilities may all be significant in selecting group members. It is important for the speech-language pathologist to assess each client's needs to decide if a group offers a reasonable solution to at least some of the variables previously described. The clinician may serve as the group leader or moderator, or may designate a member as leader. Groups may be organized for clients and/or their families and may have the same goals as individual sessions. Individual and group therapy may be scheduled in conjunction with each other, or one might be the preferred or sole format used.

Form

Direct therapy includes methods or techniques that the speech-language pathologist presents directly to clients in an attempt to improve their communication. The clinician models, teaches, stimulates, and reinforces the new behavior on the assumption that the individual recognizes that communication difficulties exist and wants to change these. With a direct format, the speech and/or language problem is "the point of attack."

Indirect therapy implies that the clinical environment is manipulated so that the new behavior evolves from the environmental changes (Leith, 1984). The practitioner helps clients discover their communication difficulties and become interested in modifying them. Counseling and family therapy are examples of indirect formats (see chapter 2 for more information about direct and indirect service delivery options).

Setting

The environment in which therapy is conducted may enhance or decrease the meaningful context of communication. The use of naturalistic formats for therapy has become increasingly popular. Clinicians and clients now work at the client's home, in the classroom, or on the playground, as well as in the traditional therapy room. By meeting clients on their own territory, the clinician can witness their responses to communication demands and to various communication partners. A major reason for the acceptance of a naturalistic format is that the clinician can attempt to structure the milieu or manipulate the environment so that it becomes a nurturing and generally helpful one in which appropriate communication behaviors are prompted. Further, the maintenance and generalization of skills across persons and settings are important therapy goals that may require a shift to varied work and social contexts. Given practical constraints, the setting still used most often seems to be the therapy room. Through attempts to adapt the clinical surroundings to the client, to construct miniclassrooms within the clinic room (see Ripich & Spinelli, 1985), and to leave our therapy rooms and enter the classroom, we are making strides toward bridging the gap between natural and clinical environments.

CONSULTATION

Definition

Consultation is an interactive process in which speech-language pathologists and audiologists assist other professionals and thereby indirectly serve individuals with communication problems. The practice of consultation includes a number of functions related to other services on the clinical spectrum. That is, consultation can be used as a form of prevention, assessment, indirect therapy, and discharge planning.

Objectives

Freeman (1985) states that "the primary purpose of professional consultation is to seek the opinion of a person with particular knowledge, information, and skills" (p. 22). The focus of consultation may differ as a result of the environment or organization in which it occurs. Obviously, the needs of physicians, attorneys, teachers, and businessmen for our professional opinions will vary. Consultations may relate to specific individuals or clients or deal with more general issues. Some goals that may remain reasonably constant include the following:

1. To assist professionals in identifying individuals with or at risk for communication problems (assessment, prevention);

2. To assist professionals in their treatment of individuals who have or are at risk for communication problems (therapy, prevention);
3. To assist professionals in establishing a diagnosis (assessment);
4. To assist professionals in developing plans or modifying activities to improve language proficiency (therapy);
5. To assist professionals in improving services to individuals with communication problems and their families;
6. To assist professionals in locating and using appropriate resources in the community (prevention, therapy, discharge planning);
7. To assist professionals in evaluating the need for and/or quality of programs and services in speech-language pathology and audiology (program assessment);
8. To assist professionals in conserving hearing, speech, and language (prevention);
9. To assist others in broadening their understanding of the profession of speech-language pathology and audiology and of individuals with communication handicaps (prevention).

Strategies

How do speech-language pathologists and audiologists satisfy these goals of consultation? There are a number of approaches or strategies that can be used. Alpert and Spencer (1986) identify a series of stages that compose the core of any consultative practice. These stages form a lucid and viable basis for approaching consultation. During the entry stage, an individual is invited to or initiates a request to serve as a consultant, and mutually acceptable goals specific to the consultee (individual or organization) are established. As an example, a speech-language pathologist might be called on to assist in modifying a phonics-based reading program for a child with a significant phonologic problem. After the preliminary contact, the speech-language pathologist and teacher might together establish clear expectations about what is to be assessed, the amount of time needed, and the best mechanism for sharing concerns.

In the second stage of the consulting process the problem or issue in question is assessed or diagnosed through careful and sensitive observation and investigation. To continue with the example just introduced, the consultant might collect information about the child, the nature of his or her speech and language problem and reading performance, the teacher, the reading program, the speech and language intervention process, and other factors so that a modification in reading instruction or alternative program can be offered.

The next step is designated as intervention and refers to the resolution of the immediate problem and an encouragement of continued consultee growth and change. At this point our case consultant might note, based on diagnostic findings, what the teacher was already doing to advance the child's reading skills and establish the child's positive attitude toward learning. The consultant might review with the teacher the child's observed strengths and weaknesses. The consultant might offer specific suggestions of materials and/or techniques that could be used to supplement the reading program within the school. Thus, intervention strategies must consider the client (here, a child with a language-based reading problem), the consultee (in this example, a teacher), and the organization (in this case, a school) (Alpert & Spencer, 1986, p. 123).

The last stage of consultation involves an evaluation of the degree to which the goals were satisfied and a termination of the consult. Referring again to our example, the consultant might wish to posttest the child with the reading problem, interview the teacher to obtain feedback, and collaborate on future plans.

Freeman (1985) observed that the three most frequent consulting activities in which school-based speech-language pathologists engage are concerned with (1) specific children and their verbal communication disorders, (2) interpretation of the profession and its relation to the local school program, and (3) materials and techniques that may be used by others to support the remedial program (p. 28). Dublinske (1970) provides examples of more than a dozen consulting services, including inservice education, case staffings, team conferences, and activities specific to a particular person. Other types of consultation programs involving speech-language pathologists include environmental assessment, expert testimony, and discharge planning. Frasinelli, Superior, and Myers (1983) offer further descriptions of consultation models for speech and language intervention. The activities suggested by these authors reflect a diverse, flexible, and potentially valuable form of intervention.

Format

The variety of strategies and activities described thus far implies that differences in consultation format exist. These differences relate to the service delivery pattern (supplementary or sole service), the consultation focus (client versus consultee), and the professional affiliations and employment arrangements.

Service Delivery Pattern

The 1983 revised report *Guidelines for Caseload Size for Speech-Language Pathology Services in the Schools* presented by the Committee on Language, Speech, and Hearing Services in the Schools (1984) includes this affirmation:

> The consultation program is not to be considered second best or to be used when direct intervention by the speech-language pathologist is not possible, but rather selection of this program should be based on the communicative needs of the student. It should be the program of choice and not of desperation. Used appropriately, this program can be most effective. Students receiving services in this program should be counted as part of the speech-language pathologist's total caseload. (p. 54)

This statement reflects a philosophy about the flexibility of the service delivery pattern of consultation. As indicated, consultations can be provided as a primary and sole service or used in conjunction with other services. The emerging acceptance of this service option is evident in the recent writing of Orme and Almerico (1986), who point out that although in the past school-based speech-language pathologists could only account for their direct services to children, today consultation is credited as a legitimate and billable procedure.

Consultation Focus

Alpert and Spencer (1986) distinguish client-centered consultation from consultee-focused services. According to these authors, the first format assesses and addresses the *client's* difficulty, whereas the second concentrates on exploring why a particular *consultee* is having difficulty with the client and how he or she may be contributing to the problem (p. 108). Consultations may involve either an individual client or a group of clients or focus on more general organizational issues.

Professional Relationships and Employment Arrangements

As discussed earlier, consultants may service professionals in their own field or work with individuals who represent another profession. Some of the professional consultations in which speech-language pathologists and audiologists engage include work with teachers, psychologists, occupational and physical therapists, physicians, attorneys, businesspeople, insurance agents, Medicare intermediaries and carriers, and personnel in Medicare regional offices and Medicaid state agencies. Thus, the consultation can occur in the schools, in industry, and in various health-care settings. The speech-language pathologist or audiologist may be hired as an internal, or in-house, consultant to work on a permanent basis or may be employed in a temporary capacity. Readers interested in more information about the nature and format of consultation in health care may wish to consult Alpert and Meyers, (1983); Caplan (1970); and Meyers, Alpert, and Fleisher (1983). The importance of consultation to speech-language pathologists and audiologists is illustrated in this statement by Flower (1984): "The single most significant indicator of our profession's growing stature and maturity may be the increasing demand for our consultative services" (p. 11).

DISCHARGE PLANNING

Definition

Over the past decade we have evidenced a period of rapid and significant change in health-care delivery. The introduction of the Medicare Prospective Payment System and the increased emphasis on utilization review and cost containment have strengthened the position of discharge planning along the service spectrum. (Refer to chapters 7 and 8 for complete information about these trends.) McKeehan (1981) suggests that "discharge planning is one of the most important elements in the delivery of health care today" (p. xiii). She defines discharge planning as "the process of activities that include the patient and a team of individuals from various disciplines working together to facilitate the transition of that patient from one environment to another" (p. 3). This description most appropriately fits discharge planning as it relates to hospitals or other health-care facilities and reflects its interdisciplinary nature. However, a speech-language pathologist or audiologist may also establish a service of discharge planning unique to a free-standing speech and hearing clinic. Within this context, discharge planning may be seen as a planned program developed and coordinated by the speech-language pathologist or audiologist to ensure that each client has the continuing or follow-up service(s) needed.

Objectives

The concept and practice of discharge planning is fairly new in speech-language pathology and audiology. However, discharge-planning models in related fields such as social work (Beck & Jones, 1980) and medicine (Hartigan & Brown, 1985; McKeehan, 1981) provide a rationale for those speech-language pathologists and audiologists responsible for integrating this service into their clinical programs. Hartigan and Brown (1985) have identified various operational functions of discharge planning. Some of the primary functions are as follows:

1. To prepare the client and family for a change in or termination of services;
2. To help arrange a shift in care from one agency or professional to another (e.g., to secure speech-language pathology services in a rehabilitation center for a patient leaving an acute-care hospital, to forward records, to prepare a new clinician);
3. To evaluate and identify current and anticipated social, emotional, and communicative needs;
4. To monitor the client's communicative status following discharge;
5. To prepare the client and family to transfer acquired skills or techniques to settings external to the original place of treatment.

The decision to discharge a client from therapy is individualized, although it is influenced to some degree by work settings, clinical philosophies, and insurer regulations. One or more of the following criteria may be considered:

1. Client has achieved therapy objectives and communication skills are judged to be acceptable.
2. Client appears to have made as much progress as physical, social/emotional, and/ or intellectual characteristics allow.
3. Client has not demonstrated commitment to therapy program in terms of attendance, completion of assignments, or overall cooperation.

4. Client is to receive services from another source (school, clinic), or needs other types of service (psychotherapy, etc.). (University of Pittsburgh Speech and Hearing Clinic, *Discharge Procedures*, 1986)

Strategies

The implementation of a discharge-planning program typically involves several strategies. First, the clinician assesses and diagnoses the severity of and prognosis for the client's communication disorder. Second, the clinician formulates and implements a discharge plan to be followed by the client, family, or other health-care provider based on the client's medical needs, family situation, transportation, insurance coverage, service options, motivation, and so forth. This may include client and family education and/or counseling to support them in assuming responsibility for continued work. Third, the clinician evaluates the discharge plan through follow-up with the client, the family, and/or a community agency serving the client. This might involve regularly scheduled phone contacts with the client or written summary notes from the present service provider. (Refer to McKeehan, 1981, and Hartigan & Brown, 1985.)

Weiner Gray (1981) describes a questionnaire used to obtain information from recipient agencies about a client's communication status following discharge. A sample of this form appears in Figure 4.1.

FIGURE 4.1 Discharge Planning and Follow-up Questionnaire

On _____, we referred the following patient, _____,
to your agency for services in the following departments: _____

So that we may better understand the continuity of services we have planned for our patient, we would appreciate your completing and returning this form

1. Did you have contact with the patient as planned?   Yes _____ No _____
2. Was the patient's condition as expected from the referral
   information?   Yes _____ No _____
3. Was this patient appropriate to your agency?   Yes _____ No _____
4. Did you experience any difficulties with this referral?
   (Explain a yes answer, please.)   Yes _____ No _____
5. Are you now continuing to provide services for this
   patient?   Yes _____ No _____

Please estimate the length of time that services will be required by the patient:

NOTE: From "Discharge Planning: A Speech-Language Pathologist's Perspective" by L. W. Gray in K. McKeehan (Ed.), *Continuing Care: A Multidisciplinary Approach to Discharge Planning*, 1981, St. Louis, MO: C. V. Mosby. Reprinted by permission.

FIGURE 4.2 Follow-up Plan

Follow-up Discontinued
Date _____
Sig. _____
(CCC-Sp Only)

I. Client's Name _____   Date of Diagnostic _____
   Birthdate _____ Age _____   Onset of Therapy _____
   Address _____   Number of Visits _____
   _____   Diagnosis _____
   Date discharge from regular therapy program effective _____
   Reason for discharge from regular therapy program _____

II. *Type of Follow-up Services Planned*

	Target Date	Comments
_____Phone Call to Client		
_____Family to Contact Clinic		
_____Re-checks		
_____Re-evaluation		
_____Referral to Other Agency		

   _____None (Give Reason) _____

   Clinician's Signature _____
   Supervisor's Signature _____

III. *Follow-up Results*
   Date of Contact _____ Type of Contact _____ Date of Next Contact _____
   Recommendations for Further Follow-up _____

   Clinician's Signature _____ Supervisor's Signature _____

   Date of Contact _____ Type of Contact _____ Date of Next Contact _____
   Recommendations for Further Follow-up _____

   Clinician's Signature _____ Supervisor's Signature _____

   Date of Contact _____ Type of Contact _____ Date of Next Contact _____
   Recommendations for Further Follow-up _____

   Clinician's Signature _____ Supervisor's Signature _____

   Date of Contact _____ Type of Contact _____ Date of Next Contact _____
   Recommendations for Further Follow-up _____

   Clinician's Signature _____ Supervisor's Signature _____

   NOTE: *Content* of contact must be summarized in a progress note.

June, 1985

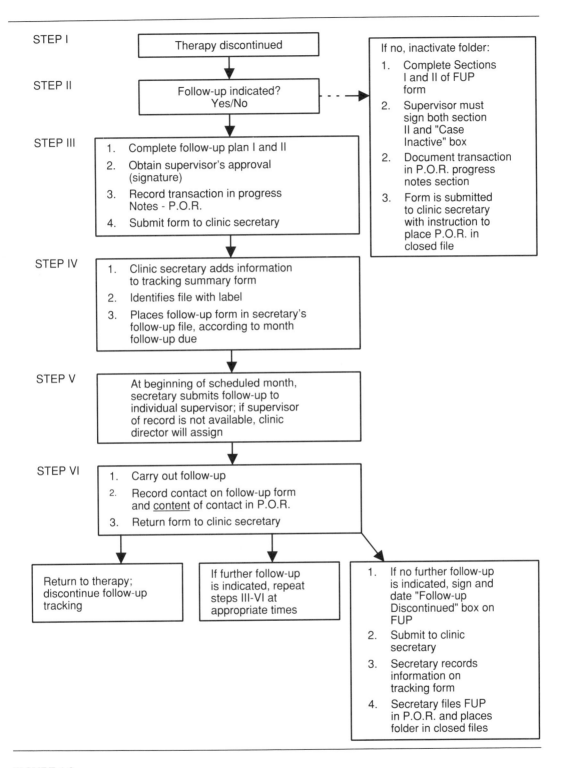

STEP I — Therapy discontinued

STEP II — Follow-up indicated? Yes/No

If no, inactivate folder:
1. Complete Sections I and II of FUP form
2. Supervisor must sign both section II and "Case Inactive" box
2. Document transaction in P.O.R. progress notes section
3. Form is submitted to clinic secretary with instruction to place P.O.R. in closed file

STEP III
1. Complete follow-up plan I and II
2. Obtain supervisor's approval (signature)
3. Record transaction in progress Notes - P.O.R.
4. Submit form to clinic secretary

STEP IV
1. Clinic secretary adds information to tracking summary form
2. Identifies file with label
3. Places follow-up form in secretary's follow-up file, according to month follow-up due

STEP V
At beginning of scheduled month, secretary submits follow-up to individual supervisor; if supervisor of record is not available, clinic director will assign

STEP VI
1. Carry out follow-up
2. Record contact on follow-up form and content of contact in P.O.R.
3. Return form to clinic secretary

Return to therapy; discontinue follow-up tracking

If further follow-up is indicated, repeat steps III-VI at appropriate times

1. If no further follow-up is indicated, sign and date "Follow-up Discontinued" box on FUP
2. Submit to clinic secretary
3. Secretary records information on tracking form
4. Secretary files FUP in P.O.R. and places folder in closed files

FIGURE 4.3
Follow-up Plan Flow Chart

NOTE: From University of Pittsburgh Speech and Hearing Clinic *Policies and Procedures Manual*, Pittsburgh, PA.

A sample of a form used at the University of Pittsburgh Speech and Hearing Clinic to document the discharge-planning process appears in Figure 4.2. This form is initiated at the time of discharge and includes the reason for termination of service and specifies the follow-up procedures indicated. A detailed Follow-up Plan (FUP) Flowchart explaining the entire procedure is provided in Figure 4.3. This system allows for an organized approach to the collection of data once regular therapy is discontinued.

Format

Weiner Gray (1981) identified options for the delivery of speech-language pathology services after the discharge of a client from a hospital. These alternatives in discharge-planning format include (1) the site where the services will be delivered (e.g., ambulatory clinic, outpatient department of a hospital, the client's home); (2) the type of service needed (e.g., group only, individual only, combination of group and individual treatment, telephone contact, probe sessions, treatment in conjunction with other health-care providers); (3) the intensity of the service required (e.g., daily, weekly, monthly); and (4) the availability of services within the client's community. Other differences in the format of discharge planning may involve the form of service (direct or indirect), and the professional affiliation of the discharge-planning coordinator (e.g., physician, nurse, psychologist, speech-language pathologist). It would seem that our longstanding concern for and interest in our clients after their discharge from therapy has promoted the development of a new clinical service. This aspect of the service spectrum, despite its relative newness, has become "a current priority" in health care (McKeehan, 1981, p. 16).

■ SUMMARY

In this chapter we have provided an overview of what speech-language pathologists do. We suggested that the key clinical services of prevention, assessment, therapy, discharge planning, and consultation are part of a spectrum in that they are ongoing, ever-changing, interactive, and at times indistinguishable processes. It seems clear that the clinical practices of speech-language pathologists are complex and challenging. We hope that the personal and professional rewards of helping individuals with communication disorders seem equally obvious.

ACTIVITIES

1. The following activity will enable you to practice description versus interpretation in clinical observation.

   Videotape your therapy session. Choose a five-minute segment of this tape. *Describe at least 20* client behaviors during the sample. Interpret all the behaviors you describe in several alternative ways, for example, see the following University of Pittsburgh class notes:

Description: *Johnny hid under the table.*
Interpretation: a) Johnny was fearful.
Interpretation: b) Johnny was concerned about the clinician's judgment.
Interpretation: c) Johnny was confused and could no longer cope with repeated requests.
Interpretation: d) Johnny was tired of endless, boring stimuli.

2. The following activity will introduce you to contingency management.

   Take half (10) behaviors your client emitted for activity 1 and do the following regarding *each* behavior:
   A. Describe the clinician's statement or act that preceded the behavior.
   B. Describe again the client's behavior that you are investigating.
   C. Interpret the client's behavior.
   D. Describe your response to your interpretation.
   E. Describe the client's response.
   F. 1. Evaluate your response sensitivity; i.e., did you respond with awareness of client motivation, or did you misinterpret?
      2. Evaluate your response consistency, i.e., did you follow the contingency program you established in advance to deal with correct, incorrect, and disruptive behaviors?

   The following are sample responses to question 2 based on University of Pittsburgh class notes.
   A. Sammy, look at the next picture.
   B. Client rested his head on the table without glancing at the picture.
   C. Client was bored by endless progression of picture stimuli.
   D. This picture has a crazy thing in it that doesn't belong there!
   E. Sammy raised his head and glanced tentatively at the picture.
   F. 1. Clinician correctly surmised that Sammy was bored and added task appeal by commenting on something unusual in the stimulus.
      2. Clinician had planned to deal with all disruptive or resistant behavior by using positive directives, i.e., appealing to what is available to the client or advising him/her of what can be earned by the next response.

3. Identify one or two other clients who might profit from group work with your client. Create three activities that might be used by this group. Remember to consider the individual communication goals for each client.

4. Observe two widely discrepant sessions and compare the different therapy approaches used.

5. Describe the two most commonly used assessment strategies at your clinic.

6. Identify one clinical strategy that may be used in at least three of the services discussed (prevention, assessment, therapy, discharge planning, or consultation). Explain how this strategy relates to these services.

7. Given your client's present needs and communication status, project an estimated discharge date and develop a discharge plan that might be implemented at that time.

8. Suppose you were asked to justify (in court, to an insurer, to your client's parents or other family members) your client's need for a particular service. Prepare a statement for this purpose.

9. Identify two prevention activities specific to speech-language pathology and/ or audiology in which you plan to engage over the next six months.

10. Identify three professionals you might consult with or invite to a staffing conference about your client.

REFERENCES

Alberto, P. A., & Troutman, A. C. (1986). *Applied behavior analysis for teachers*. Columbus, Ohio: Merrill.

Alpert, J. L., & Meyers, J. (Eds.). (1983). *Training in consultation: Mental health, behavioral, and organizational perspectives*. Springfield, IL: Charles C. Thomas.

Alpert, J. L., & Spencer, J. B. (1986). Consultation. In G. S. Tryon (Ed.), *The professional practice of psychology* (pp. 106–129). Norwood, NJ: Ablex.

ASHA Committee on Language, Speech, and Hearing Services in the Schools. (1983). Guidelines for caseload size for speech-language services in the schools. *Asha, 24*(2), 65–70.

ASHA Committee on the Prevention of Speech, Language, and Hearing Problems. (1982). Definitions of the word prevention as it relates to communicative disorders. *Asha, 24*(6), 425–431.

ASHA Committee on the Prevention of Speech, Language, and Hearing Problems. (1984). Prevention: A challenge for the profession. *Asha, 26*(8), 35–37.

ASHA Committee on the Prevention of Speech, Language, and Hearing Problems. (1984). Materials for the prevention of speech-language-hearing problems. *Asha, 26*(8), 38.

Bandura, A. (1977). *Social learning theory*. Englewood Cliffs, NJ: Prentice-Hall.

Baxter, R., Cohen, S. B., & Ylvisaker, M. (1985). Comprehensive cognitive assessment. In M. Ylvisaker (Ed.), *Head injury rehabilitation: Children and adolescents* (pp. 247–274). San Diego, CA: College-Hill Press.

Beck, D. F., & Jones, M. A. (1980). *How to conduct a client follow-up study: Some recommended procedures for local family service agencies*. New York: Family Service Association of America.

Blackstone, S. (1986). *Augmentative communication: An introduction*. Rockville, MD: ASHA.

Bloom, L. A., Johnson, C. E., Bitler, C. A., & Christman, K. L. (1986). *Facilitating communication change: An interpersonal approach to therapy and counseling*. Rockville, MD: Aspen.

Boone, D. (1971). *The voice and voice therapy*. Englewood Cliffs, NJ: Prentice-Hall.

Caplan, G. (1970). *The theory and practice of mental health consultation*. New York: Basic Books.

Carlson, F. (1981). *Alternate methods of communication: A handbook for students and clinicians.* [Sponsored by the NSSLHA.] Danville, IL: Interstate Printers and Publishers.

Cherry, L. A. (1978). A sociolinguistic approach to the study of teacher expectations. *Discourse Processes, 1*(4), 374–393.

Childrens Hospital Medical Center of Akron. (1986). Learning experience pivotal in prevention and intervention. *Special needs report, 1*(1) Akron, OH: Author.

Cook-Gumperz, J., & Gumperz, J. (1982). Communicative competence in educational perspective. In L. C. Wilkinson (Ed.), *Communicating in the classroom.* New York: Academic Press.

Courtright, J., & Courtright, I. (1976). Imitative modeling as a theoretical base for instructing language-disordered children. *Journal of Speech and Hearing Research, 19*(4), 655–663.

Dublinske, S. (1970). Consulting behavior: What-why-how. *Journal of the Iowa Speech and Hearing Association.*

Emerick, L. L., & Haynes, W. O. (1986). *Diagnosis and evaluation in speech pathology.* Englewood Cliffs, NJ: Prentice-Hall.

Fey, M. E. (1986). *Language intervention with young children.* San Diego, CA: College-Hill Press.

Flower, R. M. (1984). *Delivery of speech-language pathology and audiology services.* Baltimore, MD: Williams & Wilkins.

Frasinelli, L., Superior, K., & Myers, J. (1983). A consultation model for speech and language intervention. *Asha, 25*(1), 25–30.

Freeman, G. G. (1985). Consultation. In R. J. Van Hattum (Ed.), *Administration of speech-language services in schools* (pp. 22–53). San Diego, CA: College-Hill Press.

Gearheart, B. R. (1973). *Learning disabilities educational strategies.* St. Louis, MO: C. V. Mosby.

Goldman, R., & Dahle, A. J. (Eds.). (1985). High technology and language disorders. *Topics in Language Disorders, 6*(1).

Gray, L. W. (1981). Discharge planning: A speech-language pathologist's perspective. In K. McKeehan (Ed.), *Continuing care: A multi-disciplinary approach to discharge planning* (pp. 180–190). St. Louis, MO: C. V. Mosby.

Grossfield, M. L., & Grossfield, C. A. (Eds.). (1986). *Microcomputer applications in rehabilitation of communication disorders.* Rockville, MD: Aspen.

Haarbauer-Krupa, J., Henry, K., Szekeres, S. F., & Ylvisaker, M. (1985). Cognitive rehabilitation therapy: Late stages of recovery. In M. Ylvisaker (Ed.), *Head injury rehabilitation: Children and adolescents* (pp. 311–343). San Diego, CA: College-Hill Press.

Haarbauer-Krupa, J., Moser, L., Smith, G. J., Sullivan, D. M., & Szekeres, S. F. (1985). Cognitive rehabilitation therapy: Middle stages of recovery. In M. Ylvisaker (Ed.), *Head injury rehabilitation: Children and adolescents* (pp. 287–310). San Diego, CA: College-Hill Press.

Hartigan, E. G., & Brown, D. J. (Eds.). (1985). *Discharge planning for continuity of care.* New York: National League for Nursing.

Hegde, M. N. (1985). *Treatment procedures in communicative disorders.* San Diego, CA: College-Hill Press.

Holland, A. L. (1983). Language intervention in adults: What is it? In J. Miller, D. E. Yoder, & R. Schiefelbusch (Eds.), *Contemporary issues in language intervention* (*Asha* reports No. 12, pp. 3–13). Rockville, MD: ASHA.

Hughes, D. L. (1985). *Language treatment and generalization: A clinician's handbook.* San Diego, CA: College-Hill Press.

Jaffee, M. B., Mastrilli, J. P., Molitor, C. B., & Valko, A. S. (1985). Intervention for motor disorders. In M. Ylvisaker (Ed.), *Head injury rehabilitation: Children and adolescents* (pp. 167–194). San Diego, CA: College-Hill Press.

Katz, R. C. (1986). *Aphasia treatment and microcomputers.* San Diego, CA: College-Hill Press.

LaPointe, L. (1985) Aphasia therapy: Some principles and strategies for treatment. In D. F. Johns (Ed.), *Clinical management of neurogenic communicative disorders* (pp. 179–241). Boston: Little Brown.

Larson, V. L. & McKinley, N. L. (1987). *Communication assessment and intervention strategies for adolescents.* Eau Claire, WI: Thinking Publications.

Leith, W. R. (1984). *Handbook of clinical methods in communication disorders.* San Diego, CA: College-Hill Press.

Lund, N. J., and Duchan, J. F. (1983). *Assessing children's language in naturalistic contexts.* Englewood Cliffs, NJ: Prentice-Hall.

Marge, M. (1981). The prevention of human disabilities: Policies and practices for the 80's. In. L. G. Perlman (Ed.), *International aspects of rehabilitation: Policy guidance for the 1980s.* Alexandria, VA: National Rehabilitation Association.

——. (1984). The prevention of communication. *Asha, 26*(8), 29–33.

McCormick, L., & Schiefelbusch, R. L. (1984). *Early language intervention: An introduction.* Columbus, OH: Merrill.

McFarlane, S. C., Fujiki, M., & Brinton, B. (1984). *Coping with communicative handicaps: Resources for the practicing clinician.* San Diego, CA: College-Hill Press.

McKeehan, K. M. (Ed.). (1981). *Continuing care: A multidisciplinary approach to discharge planning.* St. Louis, MO: C. V. Mosby.

McWilliams, B. J. (1976). Various aspects of parent counseling: In E. J. Webster (Ed.), *Professional approaches with parents of handicapped children.* Springfield, IL: Charles C. Thomas.

Mehan, H. (1982). The structure of classroom events and their consequences for student performance. In P. Gilmore & A. Glatthorn (Eds.), *Children in and out of school: Ethnography and education.* Washington, DC: Center for Applied Linguistics.

Meitus, I. J. (1983). Approaching the diagnostic process. In I. J. Meitus & B. Weinberg (Eds.), *Diagnosis in speech-language pathology.* Baltimore, MD: University Park Press.

Meyers, L. F. (Ed.). (1984). Augmenting language skills with microcomputers. *Seminars in Speech and Language, 5*(1).

Meyers, J., Alpert, J. L., & Fleisher, B. D. (1983). Models of consultation. In J. L. Alpert & J. Meyers (Eds.), *Training in consultation: Mental health, behavioral, and organizational perspectives.* Springfield, IL: Charles C. Thomas.

Minifie, F. D. (1984). The personal computer as a professional tool. *Asha, 26*(6), 23–25.

Muma, J. (1978). *Language handbook: Concepts, assessment, intervention.* Englewood Cliffs, NJ: Prentice-Hall.

Nation, J. N., & Aram, D. M. (1984). *Diagnosis of speech-language disorders.* San Diego, CA: College-Hill Press.

Oliver, P., & Scott, T. (1981). Group versus individual training in establishing generalization of language skills with severely handicapped individuals. *Mental Retardation, 19,* 285–289.

Orme, D., & Almerico, B. (1986). Collaborative consultation in Jordan School District. *The Special Educator. 7*(3), 6–7.

Rees, N. S. (1978). Art and science of diagnosis in hearing, language, and speech. In S. Singh & J. Lynch (Eds.), *Diagnostic procedures in hearing, speech, and language* (pp. 3–22). Baltimore, MD: University Park Press.

Ripich, D. N., & Spinelli, F. M. (1985). An ethnographic approach to assessment and intervention. In D. N. Ripich (Ed.), *School discourse problems* (pp. 199–218). San Diego, CA: College-Hill Press.

Salvia, J., & Ysseldyke, J. E. (1978). *Assessment in special and remedial education.* Boston, MA: Houghton Mifflin.

Sanders, J. (1986). *Microcomputers and systems analysis for speech-language clinicians.* San Diego, CA: College-Hill Press.

Schultz, M. C. (1972). *An analysis of clinical behavior in speech and hearing.* Englewood Cliffs, NJ: Prentice-Hall.

Schwartz, A. H. (Ed.). (1984). *Handbook of microcomputer application in communication disorders.* San Diego, CA: College-Hill Press.

Shadden, B. B. (1987). Precrisis intervention: A tool for meeting the needs of significant others involved with aphasic older adults. *Topics in Language Disorders, 7*(3), 64–76.

Shames, G. H., & Egolf, D. B. (1976). *Operant conditioning: The management of stuttering.* Englewood Cliffs, NJ: Prentice-Hall.

Shane, H. C., & Sauer, M. (1986). *Augmentative and alternative communication.* Austin, TX: PRO-ED.

Silverman, F. H. (1987). *Microcomputers in speech-language pathology and audiology: A primer.* Englewood Cliffs, NJ: Prentice-Hall.

Spinelli, F. M., & Ripich, D. N. (1983). School discourse: How teachers, clinicians and students interact [Short course presented at the 1983 American Speech-Language-Hearing Association Meeting, Cincinnati, OH.]

Staff. (1984). Prevention: Interview with J. Michael McGinnis. *Asha, 26*(8), 22–24.

Szekeres, S. F., Ylvisaker, M., & Holland, A. L. (1985). Cognitive rehabilitation therapy: A framework for intervention. In M. Ylvisaker (Ed.), *Head injury rehabilitation: Children and adolescents* (pp. 219–246). San Diego, CA: College-Hill Press.

University of Pittsburgh Speech and Hearing Clinic. (1986). Discharge procedures and follow-up plan. *University of Pittsburgh Speech and Hearing Clinic Policies and Procedures Manual.* Pittsburgh, PA: Author.

U.S. Department of Health, Education and Welfare. (1979). *Healthy people: The surgeon general's report on health promotion and disease prevention.* Washington, DC: U.S. Government Printing Office.

Webster, E. J. (1977). *Counseling with parents and handicapped children: Guidelines for improving communication.* New York: Grune & Stratton.

Weiss, C. E., & Lillywhite, H. S. (1981). *Communicative disorders, prevention and early intervention.* St. Louis, MO: C. V. Mosby.

Weitz, J. M. (1985). An examination of classroom communication: Implications for language disordered children. Unpublished manuscript, University of Pittsburgh, Pittsburgh, PA:

Wilkinson, L. C., Clevenger, M., & Dollaghan, C. (1981). Communication in small instructional groups: A sociolinguistic approach. In W. P. Dickson (Ed.), *Children's oral communication skills* (pp. 207–240). New York: Academic Press.

Wilson, S. (1977). The use of ethnographic techniques in educational research. *Review of Educational Research, 47*(1), 245–265.

Winokur, S. (1976). *A primer of verbal behavior: An operant view.* Englewood Cliffs, NJ: Prentice-Hall.

CHAPTER FIVE

The Practice of Clinical Report Writing and Record Keeping

INTRODUCTION

This chapter may contain the most important information found in this book. Our clinical records and reports are our primary vehicles of communication with other speech-language pathologists and audiologists, health and education professionals and administrators, government agencies, and third-party payers. Patient or client records with supporting reports should provide a complete written history of the course of our work with individual patients. The accuracy and thoroughness of our documentation is often the key to third-party payment for our services and can also influence administrative decisions about the effectiveness and efficiency of our work.

For many of us, record keeping is tedious and report writing difficult, but these tasks are integral to the practice of speech-language pathology and audiology. It is our intention here to present a basic overview of documentation and reporting requirements and mechanisms commonly used in health care and public education. This generic information can be applied to a variety of situations, but it is important to determine specific requirements for content and format of records and reports in each work setting or for particular accreditation or certification agencies or payers.

CASE RECORDS

Documentation in Health Care: The Patient Record

Purposes and Contents of Health Records

The patient record is the central repository for all clinical information pertaining to an individual patient's care. Records are maintained for both inpatients and outpatients in all health-care facilities and programs. According to the Joint Commission on Accreditation of Hospitals (1986)—renamed the Joint Commission on Accreditation of Healthcare Organizations in fall 1987—the purposes of the patient (medical) record are as follows:

1. To serve as a basis for planning patient care and for continuity between evaluation and treatment;
2. To document the course of a patient's evaluation, treatment, and change in condition;
3. To document communication among health professionals who contribute to the patient's care;
4. To assist in protecting the legal interests of the patient, facility, and practitioner responsible for patient care;
5. To provide data for research, education, utilization review, and quality assurance purposes. (pp. 95–96)

Requirements for the content of patient records for individuals who receive rehabilitation services in JCAHO-accredited facilities are delineated in the *Accreditation Manual for Hospitals,* which is updated annually.

In its accreditation standards, ASHA's Professional Services Board (1984) requires that "accurate and complete records shall be prepared and maintained for each client. Records shall be accessible to appropriate personnel and systematically organized to facilitate storage and retrieval" (p. 12). According to the Board, adequate and current records are essential to the provision of quality speech-language-hearing services. PSB does not specify a particular format for case records but requires the following information:

1. Client identification data;
2. Referral source;
3. Pertinent information about the client;
4. Name of SLP/A responsible for client care;
5. Evaluation reports, treatment plans, treatment reports, and prognostic statements;
6. Chronological log of all services;
7. Dated and signed information release forms.

PSB also requires that all client records are adequately retained and "protected with respect to confidentiality, destruction, and loss" (p. 13).

Confidentiality of health information is becoming an increasingly important issue as data are computerized and used by a variety of personnel for many reasons. Most states have enacted laws that pertain to the confidentiality of information contained in patient records. Release of information usually requires the completion of an authorization form (see Appendix E), signed by the patient/ client or his or her legal representative. Authorization is not required for the review of records by health professionals currently involved in patient care, personnel who are conducting utilization review/quality assurance activities, or for certain educational and research purposes. The patient record is a legal document and may be used as evidence in legal proceedings.

In its position statement ''Confidentiality of Patient Health Information,'' the American Medical Record Association (1986) offers the following remarks regarding an individual patient's access to his or her own record:

> The health record is the physical property of the health practitioner or facility responsible for its completion. Usually, ownership of property carries with it the right and power to control the use of the property. But in the case of the health record, there is increasing recognition of the patient's right to control the information contained in his health record. The American Medical Record Association considers the health record to be the property of the health facility. The information contained in the record, however, belongs to the patient. (p. 11)

Readers should consult individual state laws and facility or program policies pertaining to confidentiality of patient records, procedures for release of information, and patient access to health records and reports.

Patient Record Formats

The Unit Record.   The unit record has been the most widely used format for recording health information in hospitals and clinics. It is a compilation of all the care provided to a single patient in a health facility. Unit records may be sectioned according to health specialty, or progress/patient-care notes may be integrated among all health-care providers. Information is presented in chronological order, and all illnesses, disorders, or problems are discussed concurrently. Flower (1984) describes the five sections of the unit record as follows:

1. application data
   (patient identification and payment information)
2. initial examination
   chief complaint
   history
   examination
   provisional diagnosis
3. progress notes
4. special examination and treatment records
   laboratory reports
   specialists' examinations and treatments
5. authorizations and correspondence (pp. 139–142)

Flower suggests an adaptation of the traditional hospital record for use in speech-language-hearing programs. This format essentially parallels the unit record but omits those portions that pertain to the needs of multiunit facilities. The adapted record includes application data, initial and reevaluations, progress notes arranged in chronological order of service, and authorizations/correspondence.

Criticisms of the unit record primarily concern the lack of a unified framework for organization of data and clinical problem solving. The chronology of information does not allow for separate focus on the components of patient illnesses or disorders. Enelow and Swisher (1979) provide a summary of their objections to the unit record:

> Information is categorized rather rigidly and arbitrarily; current findings and historical facts are usually sharply separated . . . progress notes do not commonly record an emerging synthesis and resolution of the patient's problems. Following the threads of multiple, long-term, and complex illnesses through such a record is usually a major undertaking. (p. 189)

Enelow and Swisher, among others, suggest the Problem-Oriented Record as the preferred alternative to the unit record.

The Problem-Oriented Record.   The Problem-Oriented Record (POR), developed by Weed (1968, 1969) is organized according to the patient's presenting problems. Information is referenced by separate diagnosis or components of a diagnosis and provides a focus for clinical problem solving. In multidepartmental facilities the patient's problems may be separated into medical and nonmedical diagnoses. That is, medical problems are listed and discussed in the section reserved for physicians; nonphysician health professionals address problems related to their areas of practice. PORs may also be integrated so that all health professionals address the same set of problems.

Kent and Chabon (1980), in their description of the use of the POR in a speech-language-hearing clinic, identify the four basic operations of the POR system: (1) collection of a comprehensive data base for each client; (2) identification and specification of the client's problems; (3) formulation of objectives and treatment plans; and (4) ongoing documentation of patient care. The POR format basically consists of the following elements: data base, problem list, objectives and plans, and progress notes.

The *data base* includes information pertaining to the patient's history, presenting problems, results of diagnostic evaluations, treatment reports, documents obtained from other professionals or facilities, and correspondence. It is a comprehensive core of data about the patient and the services received.

The *problem list* consists of all current problems identified through evaluation or treatment procedures, and each item must be substantiated in the data base. According to Flower (1984), "The required specific documentation of each problem, even though problems are interrelated, may be one of the greatest assets of problem-oriented records" (p. 154). Problems are modified, added, or deleted as new problems are identified, the patient makes progress, or other information becomes available.

Initial plans are prepared for each problem listed. Plans include criterion-referenced behavioral objectives which may pertain to the need to obtain further diagnostic information, treatment, and/or counseling and patient/family education. The initial plan component of the POR defines only those plans that are formulated upon the identification of a problem. Plans for continued case management are addressed in the progress-notes section.

The *progress-notes* section of the POR should provide a complete chronology of case management. Progress notes are referenced by problem number and title and are cross-referenced with items in the data base that substantiate progress-note entries or give more information (Kent & Chabon, 1980). The familiar form for POR progress notes is the "SOAP" format in which *subjective* statements about client behaviors are followed by a presentation of *objective* data, *assessment* of both subjective and objective information, and *plans* for continued treatment or evaluation. More specific information about writing progress notes is provided later in this chapter.

Problem-oriented records are originally intended for use in acute-care hospitals but have been adapted for use in many other settings (*see* Flower, 1984). The POR system is not without its critics, who point to its tendency to provide redundant information, the lack of uniform classification of problems among practitioners, and the compartmentalization of patients into "specialty zones" (Feinstein, 1973). For these reasons, Flower (1984) suggests that the POR may be best suited for "less traditional and more specialized health care delivery programs" (p. 151).

Bouchard and Shane (1977), Kovner (1984), and Frattali (1986) have praised the POR as the preferred source for gathering quality assessment and clinical research data. Other benefits of the POR for speech-language pathology and audiology programs suggested by Bouchard and Shane include ease of communication with other members of the rehabilitation team, increased efficiency in transferring client records between facilities, and facilitation of the clinical decision-making process. Refer to Bouchard and Shane (1977), Kent and Chabon (1980), and Flower (1984) for examples of POR formats and information on initiating POR systems for speech-language pathology and audiology services.

Coding Systems

Coding systems in health care were established to provide common terminology for patient diagnoses and practitioner procedures and are used for administrative, reimbursement, educational, and research purposes. Codes are recorded in patient records and on billing forms to identify the patient's illness or problem as well as the specific evaluation and treatment services rendered. Although a variety of coding systems are available for different purposes, the classifications most widely used in the United States today are the *ICD-9-CM, CPT-4,* and *DSM-III.* Our discussion will include these systems as well as two new systems that are of particular interest to speech-language pathologists and audiologists: the U.S. Public Health Service and Health Care Financing Administration Procedural

Coding System (HCPCS) and the ASHA Classification of Speech-Language Pathology and Audiology Procedures and Communication Disorders.

ICD-9-CM.   The *International Classification of Diseases, Ninth Edition (ICD-9)* was published in 1977 by the World Health Organization (WHO). It is designed for the classification of morbidity and mortality data for statistical purposes as well as for hospital-records indexing, data storage, and retrieval. The present *Clinical Modification* was published by the U.S. government in 1980 to adapt the *ICD-9* to the needs of health-care professionals and facilities in the United States. These modifications extend the basic *ICD* classifications to provide more clinical detail. The codes are published in three volumes: *Volume 1—Diseases: Tabular List; Volume 2—Diseases: Alphabetic Index;* and *Volume 3—Procedures: Tabular List and Alphabetic Index. ICD-9-CM* diseases codes are required for reporting diagnoses and diseases to all U.S. Public Health Service and Health Care Financing Administration (HCFA) programs, and this is the most widely used diagnostic coding system in the nation. The federal government maintains and updates the *ICD-9-CM* through the interdepartmental ICD-9-CM Coordination and Maintenance Committee. A 10th edition of the *International Classification of Diseases* is tentatively scheduled for publication by WHO in 1993. *Volume 3—Procedures* will not be revised at this time.

Codes used to identify communication disorders appear in the following chapters of the ninth edition:

- Chapter 5—Mental Disorders
- Chapter 6—Diseases of the Nervous System and Sense Organs
- Chapter 8—Diseases of the Respiratory System
- Chapter 14—Congenital Anomalies
- Chapter 16—Symptoms, Signs and Ill-Defined Conditions

The ICD provides a "Supplementary Classification of Factors Influencing Health Status and Contact with Health Services" (called V Codes) that are used to denote patient visits to health practitioners for purposes other than the diagnosis of a specific disease or illness. According to Flower (1984), "the V Code may be particularly useful to speech-language pathologists and audiologists since it permits the coding of client reports and presenting complaints, rather than requiring completed diagnoses" (p. 179).

Specific codes used by speech-language pathologists and audiologists are listed and discussed in Downey, White, and Karr (1984) and Flower (1984). The *ICD-9-CM* may be purchased from the U.S. Government Printing Office and is available in medical libraries and hospital medical-record departments.

CPT-4.   The *Physicians' Current Procedural Terminology, Fourth Edition (CPT-4)* is the primary system used for recording health-care services procedures in the United States. Published by the American Medical Association (AMA), the purpose of the *CPT-4* is to provide a uniform terminology that designates medical, surgical, and diagnostic services performed by physicians. The *CPT-4* first appeared in 1966 and is updated on an annual basis by the AMA.

Although the *CPT-4* is intended for use by physicians, the codes are frequently used by nonphysician health professionals as well. Speech-language pathologists and audiologists who work in health-care facilities should be familiar with the system. In addition, *CPT-4* codes are required on most health-insurance claim forms for third-party payment. A complete listing of the codes used by speech-language pathologists and audiologists appears in Flower (1984). The *CPT-4* is available for purchase from the American Medical Association.

DSM-III. The *Diagnostic and Statistical Manual of Mental Disorders, Third Edition (DSM-III)*, published by the American Psychiatric Association, is an outgrowth of the "Mental Disorders" chapter of the *ICD-9-CM*. The *DSM-III* is an expansion and modification of the ICD codes and is intended to provide further specifications for the classification of mental disorders. In addition to tabular listings in 17 categories of disorder, *DSM-III* also provides specific diagnostic criteria. Codes and descriptions related to some communication disorders are found primarily in the category "Disorders First Evident in Infancy, Childhood, or Adolescence." A complete listing of categories is found in Downey, White, and Karr (1984) and Flower (1984). Flower also delineates the diagnostic criteria for mental retardation, stuttering, developmental reading disorder, developmental receptive and expressive language disorders, and developmental articulation disorder. According to Downey, White, and Karr (1984):

> The inclusion of speech, language, and hearing disorders in the DSM-III promotes diagnosis of communicative disorders by psychiatrists more than does the ICD-9-CM . . . the manual does not accurately represent communication disorders . . . In most instances the actual codes are identical to the ICD-9-CM codes and could be used when filing a claim calling for the use of the DSM-III. This might be the case if the coverage were included under a mental disorders benefit. (p. IV–76)

It should be noted, however, that speech-language pathologists who work in psychiatric facilities may be required to use *DSM-III* codes.

HCPCS. The HCFA (Health Care Financing Administration) Common Procedure Coding System (HCPCS) was developed to satisfy the operational needs of the Medicare and Medicaid fee-for-service reimbursement programs by replacing the variety of coding systems in use with a single national reimbursement coding system. HCPCS codes are based upon the *CPT-4*, but additional codes and modifiers were developed specifically for use by nonphysician health professionals and insurers. HCFA publishes the codes in both hard copy and magnetic tape for use by health-facilities personnel, Medicare carriers, and state Medicaid agencies with certified Medical Management Information Systems (MMIS). In addition to procedure codes, HCPCS provides revenue codes for ancillary services such as pharmacy, physical therapy, and speech-language pathology.

As of July 1, 1987, HCFA required the use of HCPCS codes for all hospital outpatient surgery and laboratory services rendered under the Medicare and Medicaid programs. HCPCS replaced the *ICD-9-CM* procedure codes for those services only. According to HCFA officials, the use of HCPCS is currently experimental. Its expansion will depend upon the results of data analysis. HCFA hopes to use HCPCS to build a data base for implementing a Prospective Payment System for outpatient services for participants in government health programs.

ASHACS.   The American Speech-Language-Hearing Association Classification of Speech-Language Pathology and Audiology Procedures and Communication Disorders (ASHACS) was approved by ASHA in 1987. Developed by the Task Force on Classification Systems, ASHACS is intended for use by speech-language pathologists and audiologists in all practice settings. It provides a standard nomenclature with which to identify communication disorders and the evaluation and treatment services rendered by speech-language pathologists and audiologists. The ASHACS document states:

> The classification of speech-language pathology and audiology procedures and disorders of human communication into a numerical coding system will permit diverse, comprehensive analysis of professional services data. Uniformity of nomenclature allows review of procedures performed and disorders identified within professional settings as well as among a population of service providers. The incidence of a communication disorder in different geographical regions and the type of treatment used can also be examined. The classifications are independent of medical coding systems and assure the provision of autonomous judgment by the speech-language pathologist and audiologist. (p. 1)

The codes are divided into the following categories:

- Speech-Language Pathology and Audiology Procedures (procedures common to both areas of practice)
- Audiologic Procedures
- Speech-Language Pathology Procedures
- Speech, Language and Related Diagnoses
- Auditory and Other Diagnoses

ASHA is encouraging the inclusion of its classification system in whole or in part in some of the major coding systems and its recognition by health insurance companies for reimbursement purposes. ASHACS is incorporated into the ASHA Program Evaluation System (see chapter 8) and is also available by contacting the American Speech-Language-Hearing Association.

Documentation in Public Education: The Individual Education Program (IEP)

Our country's public education system experienced major changes in documentation requirements for special education services with the enactment of the Education for All Handicapped Children Act of 1975 (PL 94–142). These requirements provide a uniform framework for accountability that the health-care system has not yet developed, and we focus now on the central component of PL 94–142: the Individualized Education Program (IEP).

Content of the IEP

Public Law 94–142 established specific requirements for assuring that all handicapped children receive a "free, appropriate education in the least restrictive environment." The Individualized Education Program (IEP) is a written statement designed as the central mechanism by which the provisions of the law are documented. An IEP must be established and maintained for each child who participates in special education programs.

IEPs should record all programs, services, methods, equipment, and materials that are necessary to provide an appropriate education for each handicapped child. The IEP can also be a valuable tool in assessing the quality of services as well as the effectiveness of specific remedial approaches. According to Dublinske (1978), "The primary reason for . . . developing an IEP is to record that information needed to make decisions regarding the direction a handicapped child's educational program should take" (p. 382).

The required content of the IEP, as outlined in the U.S. Code of Federal Regulations (34 CFR–1985), is as follows:

a. a statement of the child's present levels of educational performance;
b. a statement of annual goals, including short-term instructional objectives;
c. a statement of the specific special education and related services to be provided to the child, and the extent to which the child will be able to participate in regular educational programs;
d. the projected dates for initiation of services and the anticipated duration of the services; and
e. appropriate objective criteria and evaluation procedures and schedules for determining, on at least an annual basis, whether the short-term instructional objectives are being achieved. (p. 80)

State education agencies may require that additional information be included in the IEP. Other pertinent data suggested by Turnbull, Strickland, and Brantley (1982) include a procedural checklist, student's schedule, a list of IEP committee members, relevant test information, student health status, special materials needed, and the specifying of persons responsible for teaching the objectives. The required format for the IEP varies among state and local education agencies. Sample formats are illustrated in Dublinske (1978), Nelson (1979), and Turnbull, Strickland, and Brantley (1982), as well as many other publications.

Development of the IEP

IEPs are developed according to a prescribed placement process which begins with a referral and extends through the Individualized Education Program Committee (IEPC) meeting. An outline of the placement process appears in Figure 5.1. *Referrals* for possible evaluation may come from any source, including physicians, school personnel, parents, students, and representatives of other agencies. Written *parental* consent must be obtained prior to the preplacement

FIGURE 5.1
The IEP Process

1. Referral
2. Obtain written parental consent to evaluate
3. Appoint multidisciplinary evaluation team (MET)
4. Conduct comprehensive evaluation
5. Team reports evaluation results
6. Inform parents of evaluation findings
7. Hold IEPC meeting
   a. Determine the student's eligibility for special education
   b. Develop IEP
   c. Obtain parents' consent to place child in special education
8. Implement IEP—one year
9. IEP annual review
10. Three-year reevaluation

evaluation. If parents refuse, or do not respond to repeated attempts to obtain consent, the school district may resolve the issue through due process procedures. (Due process will be explained later in this discussion.) The *preplacement evaluation* must be conducted by a multidisciplinary evaluation team (MET). (See chapter 6 for a description of requirements pertaining to this team.) After the evaluation, team members issue written reports of their findings. Parents must be informed of the results of the evaluation. An *IEP committee meeting* is then scheduled to determine the appropriate placement for the student. Participants in this meeting must include:

1. The child's classroom teacher;
2. A representative of the public agency who is qualified to provide or supervise special education;
3. The child's parent (or legal guardian or surrogate parent);
4. The student, when appropriate;
5. Other individuals at the request of the parent or agency;
6. The person who conducted the student's evaluation or a person knowledgeable in the interpretation of evaluation data (if the student is being considered for initial special education placement).

The placement committee is charged with determining the educational placement for the child that will result in the provision of appropriate educational services in the least restrictive environment. This means that agency personnel must facilitate the student's participation in regular education activities as much as the child's handicap will allow.

The special education student's IEP is implemented for one year from the start of services. A review of the IEP is conducted at least annually by the IEP committee for each handicapped child. The IEP is modified according to the student's achievement of annual goals and objectives. The new IEP is implemented for the next one-year cycle. Every three years a reevaluation must be administered to determine the student's continuing eligibility for special education services.

Although the IEP is used as a compliance-monitoring-evaluation document, federal regulations stress that the IEP is not a "performance document." Special education personnel are not held accountable, per se, if a child does not achieve the specific annual goals projected in the IEP. However, personnel should make every attempt to facilitate achievement of stated objectives. The success of the IEP may often depend upon the feasibility of the goals and objectives chosen by personnel. Turnbull, Strickland, and Brantley (1982) offer a checklist to assist individuals in assessing and documenting the appropriateness of the IEP with respect to legal requirements as well as relevance, manageability, and clarity of goals, objectives, and special education services. This checklist is reprinted in Figure 5.2.

Due Process

The due process system is intended to assure all parties that a child is receiving or will receive the appropriate educational services. Due process consists of procedural safeguards that protect both the state and parents with regard to the program-placement process. The following procedures are usually included:

1. A written notice must be given to parents before any action is taken or recommended that may affect the child's placement.
2. Parents have a right to examine all records related to identification, evaluation, or placement of a child.
3. Parents may register a complaint and request a meeting with educational personnel to resolve differences about a child's placement.
4. Parents have a right to obtain an independent educational evaluation at public expense if they disagree with the findings of the assessment team. However, states have specific procedures that must be followed in obtaining approval for such evaluations.
5. An impartial hearing before a hearing officer or judge must be provided if school personnel and parents/guardians cannot resolve differences of opinion.
6. An appeals procedure must be instituted if the parent or the school is not satisfied with the outcome of the hearing. The case may reach the state department of education or the civil courts.

Readers are referred to Dublinske and Healey (1978) and Turnbull, Strickland, and Brantley (1982) for detailed discussions about due process.

FIGURE 5.2
Checklist for Documenting Appropriateness of the IEP

Student Name _____

Date of Committee Meeting _____

Committee Chairperson _____

	Yes	No	Comments
Legal Requirements			
1. Does plan include all information required by law?			
a. level of performance			
b. annual goals			
c. short-term instructional objectives			
d. schedules of evaluation			
e. procedures for evaluation			
f. related services			
g. specific special education			
h. extent of participation in the regular classroom			
i. projected dates for initiation and duration of services			
Relevance			
1. Are goals, objectives, evaluation procedures, placement, and services:			
a. appropriate to the handicap of the student?			
b. determined in consideration of identified strengths and weaknesses?			
c. appropriate to the student's level of performance?			
2. Are the specified evaluation procedures correlated with the goals and objectives?			
3. Do the minimum acceptable criteria stated in objectives seem realistic for the student?			
Manageability			
1. Is the anticipated progress proportional to the amount of instructional time available?			
2. Are the procedures scheduled for evaluation reasonable considering the time and methods involved?			
3. Has the method for provision of related services been determined?			
Clarity			
1. Is the terminology used in the plan understandable to all other committee members?			
2. Is the student's level of performance specified in terms of specific skill statements?			
3. Do short-term instructional objectives clearly state:			
a. the specific behavior to be required of the student?			
b. the condition under which the behavior is to occur?			
c. the minimum acceptable criteria for attaining the objectives?			

FIGURE 5.2 *Continued*
Checklist for Documenting Appropriateness of the IEP

4. Do annual goals indicate what the student will be able to do when the IEP is terminated?
5. Do evaluation procedures specify the type of evaluation to be used and, where appropriate, specific tests?
6. Does the schedule of evaluation clearly indicate how often evaluation will occur?
7. Is the special education to be provided stated in specific terms?
8. Are related services clearly specified in terms of extent or amount of services to be provided?

NOTE: From Developing and Implementing Individualized Education Programs, by A. Turnbull, B. Strickland, and J. Brantley, 1982, Columbus, OH: Merrill. Copyright 1982 by Merrill. Reprinted with permission.

THE FORMS OF COMMUNICATION

Communication about the client by the professional takes many forms. The scope of this communication may depend on the particular client, the nature and complexity of his or her problem, the need for rapid conveyance of information, and the service setting. In this section, we describe several forms of communication used by speech-language pathologists, including clinical reports, letters and administrative authorizations, and staffings.

Clinical Reports

Assessment is typically initiated during a client's first visit to the speech and hearing clinic and is documented in a *diagnostic report* or case report. Emerick and Haynes (1986) offer this definition of a diagnostic report:

> [It] is a written record that summarizes the relevant information we have obtained and 'how' we have obtained it in our professional interaction with a client. It serves the following function:
> 1. It acts as a guide for further services to the client providing a clear statement of how the person was functioning at a given point in time, so that we can document change or lack of change;
> 2. It communicates our findings to other professional workers; it provides answers to a number of clinical questions, including: Does the person have a problem? How severe is the problem? Will therapy be helpful? and
> 3. It serves as a document for research purposes. (p. 318)

Diagnostic reports are a form of communication that may assume varied formats. Despite some inconsistencies in definition, there are several essential elements of a diagnostic report. These elements are discussed in the accompanying box.

ESSENTIAL ELEMENTS OF A DIAGNOSTIC REPORT

Identifying data include the client's name, address, telephone number, birthdate and/or age, sex, date of assessment, and referral source. This information may be collected at the time of the assessment or abstracted from the case history questionnaire after verbal confirmation of its accuracy from the client or informant.

A *statement of the problem* summarizes the client's "chief complaint" or referral agent's primary concern. The focus here is on the client's description of the problem and the reasons for seeking assistance at the time. This statement often includes exact quotations from the content of the client interview as well as material from earlier evaluations.

Background information is obtained from a case-history questionnaire, interviews, and referral letters and includes descriptions of the family constellation and home environment, medical, developmental, social-educational histories, and previous intervention efforts. Although all aspects of development are reviewed, speech and language acquisition are likely to receive special attention.

Test results and observations relevant to the client's communication are described. The extend and specificity of this description will depend on the purpose of the evaluation and of the report (Flower, 1984, p. 104). Those aspects of communication that were not the focus of the complaint and were found to be age appropriate or unremarkable or were not assessed due to noncompliance or time limitations should be discussed briefly.

In the *clinical impressions* section of the report the practitioner expresses his or her clinical opinion about the correlates or causes of the presenting problem, interprets assessment findings, describes the client's assets and deficits (Pannbacker, 1975), and establishes a prognosis. According to Meitus (1983), the clinical impression is the formulation of a diagnosis.

Through *recommendations* the practitioner translates the diagnostic data into suggestions about what to do. They should be supported by the objective and subjective assessment findings. Some clinicians prefer to write statements that specify the frequency and nature of treatment. If therapy will be provided by the same individual or at that same facility, this may be ideal. On the other hand, detailed and unequivocal recommendations may be difficult to implement as proposed by another clinician at a different facility and may create confusion on the part of clinicians and clients alike. This point is addressed by Emerick and Haynes (1986), who believe that the recommendations should "provide a flexible blueprint for further action" (p. 324).

All diagnostic reports should be signed by the responsible diagnostician and carry his or her title and professional qualifications (e.g., license or certification status). If these individuals are not certified in speech-language pathology, the report should ideally be cosigned by a certified clinician. See Appendix F for a sample diagnostic report format. This structure can be easily adapted to different clinical settings and allows the information to be organized so that it can be readily understood. Depending on the nature of the referral, the focus of the assessment, and the particular work place, certain sections may receive more emphasis and some may even be excluded.

Diagnostic reports should be completed, filed in the client's record, and disseminated to authorized individuals within 15 working days after completion of the evaluation. The clinician may wish to explain verbally the contents of the report to the parents, client, or teacher or prepare a summary statement based on this more complete document.

Therapy Plans and Flowcharts

A therapy plan, or educational plan, details the objectives and procedures relevant to a particular client during a specified therapy period. It may cover one session or extend over a longer period of time. A therapy plan may be structured as a flowchart or be used as a data sheet on which to tabulate a client's responses alongside stated goals. Flower (1984) points out that a therapy plan may comprise one section of an evaluation report or be written as a separate report.

University-based training clinics often require that students complete a therapy plan prior to each session. Typically this plan must be approved by a clinical supervisor before procedures can be implemented. More experienced clinicians may not always utilize this approach, although third-party payers such as Medicaid and Medicare, and accrediting agencies such as the Joint Commission on Accredition of Healthcare Organizations (JCAHO) and the Professional Services Board (PSB) require documentation of therapy plans.

Examples of therapy plans include the IEP, which is associated with school programs, and problem-oriented records, which are linked with hospitals and other health-care facilities. Although the specificity in content and the structure of the plan vary greatly, a few elements remain reasonably constant. Behavioral objectives, which are time- and criterion-referenced plans for achieving these goals, are often included. Behavioral objectives are goal statements that identify in precise behavioral terms what a client is expected to do, under what circumstances and for how long, and the criterion level for goal modification. Procedures refer to what the clinician will do to elicit the response. This includes the specific techniques, tasks, materials, and method of reinforcement used to achieve goals. These descriptions may be accompanied by a statement of rationale or reason for doing a procedure. The plan may also be used as a data sheet for recording the client's responses (Kent & Chabon, 1980). See appendixes G and H for samples of lesson-plan formats.

Progress Notes and Summary Progress Reports

Progress notes are a form of report required on a regular or at least periodic basis in most work settings; therefore, such notes represent a significant aspect of the communication process. Progress notes serve as documentation of the therapy plan, the course and outcome of therapy, and the delivery of services (Kent & Chabon, 1980). Progress notes provide a complete and continuous record of all contacts (e.g., phone calls, letters, observations, therapy services, cancellations, clients' expressions of satisfaction or complaints about therapy, clinicians' suggestions or referrals) with or on behalf of the client. These entries are usually titled to distinguish the type of contact being documented (e.g., phone contact versus therapy session). Some progress notes are appropriately short, whereas others may consist of detailed descriptions of therapy events.

Knepflar (1976) outlined three features of good progress notes:

1. Brief notes concerning specific clinical management techniques and materials used.
2. Interpretation of how the patient responded and statements regarding the patient's progress.
3. Suggestions or assignments given to the patient and, when appropriate, recommendations for the next session. (p. 23)

Progress notes are generally characterized as either of two types: narrative (SOAP note) and flow sheets (diagrammatic and graphic). SOAP, an acronym for subjective-objective-assessment-plan, was discussed earlier in this chapter. Appendix I contains an example of a simple form that can be used for such reports. Flow sheets or graphic notes are typically charts used to record and monitor measurable behaviors from one session to the next. The Base-10 Response Form available through Pro-Ed of Austin, Texas, is one example (LaPointe, L. [1987–88 catalog]. *Base-10 Response Form.* Austin, TX: Pro-Ed.)

Hollis and Donn (1979) describe a third type of progress note written by the clinician in an informal manner for his or her personal use. These notes may include direct quotes of statements made by the client, comments on the client's appearance and behavior during the session, or explanations of the clinician's responses, procedures, and so forth (p. 156). Typically, these notes are highly confidential and not shared with others, unless required by law.

In addition to regular progress notes a periodic summary progress report may be required. This report, as its name suggests, summarizes the events of treatment as recorded in the progress notes over a certain period of time. Summary progress reports enable the clinician to monitor the quality of service to clients and assess the effectiveness of treatment plans. Knepflar (1976) states that "summary reports should always include statements regarding specific clinical approaches, methods or techniques that were particularly successful with a patient . . . (as well as) those that were met with resistance or rejection by a patient" (p. 24). A sample outline for the summary progress report is included in Appendix J. All progress-note entries and summary reports should be signed by their authors.

Discharge Summaries and Referrals

Discharge summaries serve several important functions: (1) to facilitate the continuity of care when a client is transferred from one clinician to another, or from one facility to another, or when requests for authorization of additional services are made; (2) to uphold standards of quality "through protection of accreditation, maintenance of supervisory control and compliance with laws affecting the defense of a claim" (Gray, 1981, p. 176); (3) to encourage the review or coordination of a total rehabilitation program by the original referring agent (Flower, 1984); and (4) to facilitate easy access to information about the nature and effects of therapy for use in research or further service. Flower contends that discharge summaries should be mandatory regardless of the reasons for termination of therapy.

According to Gray (1981), discharge summaries should contain the following information:

1. Client identification data.
2. Client's course of treatment and response to it.
3. Indications and contraindications to therapy and functional abilities.
4. Functional status at discharge (including the client's physical status as it relates to abilities and limitations).
5. Goals initially established and those achieved at discharge (including reasons for not meeting some goals).
6. Discharge plans (placement, level of care required, home program, assistance of family and support systems, equipment required, etc.). (p. 176)

This author distinguishes discharge summaries from referral forms. She describes referral writing as "a synopsis of the discharge summary" and suggests that it contains fewer specific details on the course and outcome of therapy. Thus, the discharge summary supports the referral process and accompanies the referral document.

The referral form itself should, minimally, clarify the reasons for the referral and the expectations or specific requests of the person or agency initiating the referral. The exact content will vary with the purpose of the referral and the level of sophistication of the individual to whom the referral is being addressed. A basic principle of any referral procedure is that it be thorough and clear. Appendix K includes an example of a referral form used to communicate referrals to otolaryngologists about individuals with voice disorders. It states clearly the specific questions to be answered by this specialist.

Letters

King and Berger (1971) describe a good letter as one that accomplishes its purpose. Indeed, letter writing in speech-language pathology serves many and varied purposes. Some of these goals have been accounted for as reports and include making referrals, preparing progress notes, and developing closing statements or discharge summaries. Others most often take the form of letters and involve requesting information about a client; requesting authorization to release or obtain information about a client, to use data that belong to another person, or to engage the client in a particular activity (e.g., permit audio- or videotaping of a session); acknowledging receipt of referrals; confirming appointments; and notifying clients of a change in clinic policy (e.g., increase in fees) or a need to adhere to current policy (e.g., terminate therapy due to irregular attendance). Copies of all correspondence should be maintained in the client records. Notation of these transactions in the progress notes is also recommended. The specific format of these written communications is less important than their clarity and accuracy. Sample letters and descriptive outlines from the fields of speech-language pathology, psychology, and remedial reading can be found in Meitus (1983), Hollis and Donn (1979), and Rude and Oehlkers (1984). Your own clinic's case folders are most likely to contain a wealth of exemplary materials suitable to that particular setting. A few examples of letters we have utilized successfully in clinical practice are provided in appendixes L and M.

Case Staffings and Team Conferences

The case staffing, or team conference, is a client-centered meeting at which those individuals involved with a particular case convene to discuss treatment goals and evaluate the delivery of care. This conference provides a mechanism for clinical management, professional interaction, and staff development. In terms of clinical management, the team reports on the status of and/or need for speech-language therapy, comments on it, and suggests possible variations or supports continuation of the therapy plan. Public Law 94–142 requires a multidisciplinary staffing before a child may be placed in a special education program. Professional interaction is facilitated by a staffing because its success depends on the involvement of each member of the team. Staff development is promoted through the sharing of interdisciplinary information.

All clients should be staffed as part of a clinician's commitment to the processes of continuity of care and to the assessment of the quality of care. Some facilities have established predetermined guidelines as to when in the clinical process a client is to be staffed or a team conference held. Other agencies have identified staffing priorities such as the development of long- and short-term goals immediately after assessment; identification of specific problems with or questions about clinical management; demonstration of a unique approach to or experimental model of therapy; consideration for termination of treatment; and follow-up review of clients previously dismissed from therapy. The timing of a team conference will vary according to its primary purpose and in relation to the nature of the work setting. For example, IEP conferences are usually conducted soon after a problem has been identified. Rehabilitation team conferences may be held on a regular (e.g., weekly) basis throughout a client's stay.

A staffing is usually structured to include a report about the pertinent case-history data, diagnostic information, date therapy was initiated, cumulative number of sessions, specific intervention method used, progress observed, and future plans. Our personal experience suggests that these discussions may be enhanced by using video- or audiotapes of client behavior, inviting consultants or other professionals who are directly involved with the client, allowing time for discussion and questions, and recording impressions and recommendations in progress notes or final summary progress reports. In summary, staffings afford the optimal setting for the exchange of observations and insights among the members of various disciplines for the benefit of the client but also for the immediate enlightenment and long-term education of the members of the group.

Obviously, written communications are an important part of all of the forms of professional assessment and interaction we have discussed in this section—from clinical reports to team conferences. In discussing the process of writing, Emerick and Haynes (1986) observe that

> Many students have difficulty writing reports. Most of them have found the task onerous, and few are threatened and overwhelmed by the prospect of a blank sheet of paper in the typewriter. . . However . . . rather than a writing 'deficiency' most of these students have a writing 'bias'—they do not think they can do it. (p. 329)

Similarly, Haynes and Hartman (1975) comment about "the agony of report writing" from their personal experiences as students and as supervisors by noting that:

> [These reports] are a major source of conflict, negative emotion and student insecurity. Each quarter in universities across the country, there exists a massive ebb and flow of clinical reports between supervisors and student clinicians. The reports are submitted to the supervisors and then returned to the students with numerous multicolored criticisms. These flaws must then be corrected and the reports resubmitted to the supervisor for further scrutiny. So it goes, back and forth. In many cases, the report goes through this process so repeatedly that the finished product is almost totally written in installments by the supervisor. The reasons behind the supervisor's manifold revisions are not always clear to the burgeoning speech clinician; however, these students are assured that they will understand the rationale and substance of the corrections when they have had more experience with report writing. (p. 7)

These accounts suggest a practice and a perspective prevalent in the clinical education of students in the art and science of clinical report writing.

■ SUMMARY

In this chapter we have presented the essentials of professional communication. Health data needs will continue to increase as the health-care system focuses on controlling costs, utilization, and quality of services. Documentation and coding requirements will likely become more standardized within health professions, especially as data are converted to automated management information systems. The speech-language pathology and audiology profession is keeping pace with these developments with the introduction of ASHA's Classification of Speech-Language Pathology and Audiology Procedures and Communication Disorders as well as its computerized Program Evaluation System. We will continue to be challenged, however, by new data requirements and technological innovations as the health-care system continues its rapid change and refinement.

In this chapter we briefly described the IEP and its centrality to the Education for All Handicapped Children Act (PL 94–142). Speech-language pathologists and audiologists who work in schools must be knowledgeable about federal, state, and local education-agency requirements that apply to the development of IEPs as well as provision of services to handicapped children. The IEP is integral to the comprehensive program-planning, implementation, and evaluation process required by PL 94–142. Dublinske (1978) maintains that "the IEP concept provides speech-language pathologists and audiologists with a unique opportunity and responsibility . . . to see that the IEP is used appropriately and to advantage in improving the quality of education for handicapped children" (p. 383). The IEP, then, is the primary accountability mechanism for ensuring that the individual educational needs of handicapped children are met.

As specialists in human communication and its disorders, speech-language pathologists and audiologists should describe and document their work with clarity and precision. A well-written report or letter, or a concisely presented case staffing, can only enhance the practitioner's professional image. More importantly, documentation is the primary basis for making judgments about the quality of our services. In addition, decisions about appropriate utilization of and payment for services rendered are usually made after reviewing records and reports. The importance of developing excellent professional communication skills cannot be overemphasized. Although it is not an easy task for most of us, it is one investment in which the dividends are assured.

ACTIVITIES

1. Survey speech-language-hearing programs in your area to determine what client record systems are being used. Devise a series of questions to ask clinic or program directors about their record-keeping systems. In addition, ask about what numerical coding systems (e.g., ICD, DSM, CPT, HCPCS, ASHACS, or others) are used.

2. Using one (or more) of the coding systems identified in this chapter, code the diagnosis for each of your clients as well as the procedures used for evaluation and treatment.

3. If your clinic does not use the POR, formulate a problem list for each of your clients.

4. Write SOAP progress notes for the identified problems.

5. Obtain your state's requirements for implementation of PL 94–142. If you plan to work in the schools in another state, write for that state's regulations. Note: Even if you do not plan a career as a school practitioner, it is important to be familiar with the regulations. You may be asked to provide an independent evaluation, appear as an expert witness at a due process hearing, or otherwise assist in formulating or revising an Individualized Education Program (IEP).

6. Obtain a sample IEP form. Complete an IEP for a child whose primary handicap is a speech or language impairment.

7. Prepare a speech-language-hearing discharge summary outline for use in one or more of the following practice settings: acute-care hospital, rehabilitation hospital, home-care agency, community clinic.

8. Write a sample referral letter to a physician, psychologist, or occupational therapist.

9. Observe a case staffing in your clinic, then plan a case staffing for one of your clients.

10. Write a critique of the record and reporting system used in a clinic or program in which you participate. Prepare a set of recommendations for improving the system.

REFERENCES

American Medical Association. (1986). *Physicians' current procedural terminology* (4th ed.) *(CPT-4)*. Chicago, IL: American Medical Association.

American Medical Record Association. (1986). *Confidentiality of patient health information.* Chicago, IL: AMRA.

American Psychiatric Association. (1980). *Diagnostic and statistical manual of mental disorders* (3rd ed.) *(DSM-III)*. Washington, DC: American Psychiatric Press.

ASHA. (1987). *The American Speech-Language-Hearing Association classification of speech-language pathology and audiology procedures and communication disorders.* Rockville, MD: ASHA.

ASHA, Professional Services Board. (1984). *Accreditation manual.* Rockville, MD: ASHA.

Bouchard, M., & Shane, H. (1977). Use of the problem-oriented medical record in the speech and hearing profession. *Asha, 19*(3), 157–159.

Downey, M., White, S., & Karr, S. (1984). *Health insurance manual for speech-language pathologists and audiologists.* Rockville, MD: ASHA.

Dublinske, S. (1978). PL 94–142: Developing the individualized education program (IEP). *Asha, 20*(5), 380–397.

Dublinske, S., & Healey, W. (1978). PL 94–142: Questions and answers for the speech-language pathologist and audiologist. *Asha, 20*(3), 188–205.

Emerick, L., & Haynes, W. (1986). *Diagnosis and evaluation in speech pathology* (3rd ed.). Englewood Cliffs, NJ: Prentice-Hall.

Enelow, A., & Swisher, S. (1979). *Interviewing and patient care.* New York: Oxford University Press.

Feinstein, A. (1973). The problems of the 'problem-oriented medical records.' *Annals of Internal Medicine, 78,* 751–762.

Flower, R. (1984). *Delivery of speech-language pathology and audiology services.* Baltimore, MD: Williams & Wilkins.

Frattali, C. (1986, May). Are we reaching our goals? Developing outcome measures. In P. Larkins (Ed.), *In search of quality assurance: What lies ahead?* [ASHA Quality Assurance Workshop Manual]. Rockville, MD: ASHA.

Gray, L. (1981). Discharge planning: A speech-language pathologist's perspective. In K. McKeehan (Ed.), *Continuing care: A multidisciplinary approach to discharge planning* (pp. 180–190). St. Louis, MO: Mosby.

Haynes, W., & Hartman, D. (1975). The agony of report writing: A new look at an old problem. *Journal of the National Student Speech and Hearing Association, 3*(1), 7–15.

Hollis, J., & Donn, P. (1979). *Psychological report writing: Theory and practice.* Muncie, IN: Accelerated Development.

Joint Commission on Accreditation of Hospitals. (1986). *Accreditation manual for hospitals/87.* Chicago, IL: JCAH.

Kent, L., & Chabon, S. (1980). Problem-oriented record in a university speech and hearing clinic. *Asha, 22*(3), 151–158.

King, R., & Berger, K. (1971). *Diagnostic assessment and counseling techniques for speech-language pathologists and audiologists.* Pittsburgh, PA: Stanwix House.

Knepflar, K. (1976). *Report writing in the field of communication disorders.* Danville, IL: Printers & Publishers.

Kovner, C. (1984). Quality assurance and the patient record. In J. Pena et al. (Eds.), *Hospital quality assurance* (pp. 207–217). Rockville, MD: Aspen Systems.

Meitus, I. (1983). Clinical report and letter writing. In I. Meitus & B. Weinberg (Eds.), *Diagnosis in speech-language pathology* (pp. 1–30). Baltimore, MD: University Park Press.

Nelson, N. (1979). *Planning individualized speech and language intervention programs.* Tucson, AZ: Communication Skill Builders.

Pannbacker, M. (1975). Diagnostic report writing. *Journal of Speech and Hearing Disorders, 40*(3), 367–379.

Rude, R., & Oehlkers, W. (1984). *Helping students with reading problems.* Englewood Cliffs, NJ: Prentice-Hall.

Turnbull, A., Strickland, B., & Brantley, J. (1982). *Developing and implementing individual education programs.* Columbus, OH: Merrill.

U.S. Department of Health and Human Services, Health Care Financing Administration. (1980). *International classification of diseases* (9th ed.), *Clinical modification (ICD-9-CM)* (DHHS Publication No. PHS 80–1260). Washington, DC: U.S. Government Printing Office.

U.S. Office of the Federal Register. (1985). *Code of federal regulations.* Washington, DC: U.S. Government Printing Office.

Weed, L. (1968). Medical records that guide and teach. *New England Journal of Medicine, 278,* 652–657.

———. (1969). *Medical records, medical education and patient care: The problem-oriented record as a basic tool.* Cleveland, OH: Case Western Reserve University.

CHAPTER SIX

Working with Other Professionals

INTRODUCTION

Speech-language pathology services are part of a complex and interdependent health-care delivery system. There are many health professionals who provide highly specialized services to patients of all ages whose health-care needs vary widely. For some speech-language pathologists, contact with other professionals is very limited. Others have daily team treatment sessions that involve two or three other professionals. Team staffings may include perhaps 2 to 10 professional or technical personnel. We belive that effective interprofessional relationships, and ultimately patient care, are facilitated by the quality of our knowledge about the credentials, responsibilities, and contributions of other professionals to the team process.

WHO ARE OTHER PROFESSIONALS?

The following descriptions are intended to provide a brief overview of the professionals with whom speech-language pathologists commonly interact: physicians, nurses, physical therapists, occupational therapists, psychologists, social workers, and educators. It is by no means an exhaustive list. As you read the descriptions, think about how each professional contributes to patient care. In later sections we discuss the practical aspects of working with other professionals, including potential sources of conflict as well as exciting trends in team approaches to service delivery.

Physicians

We all have an opinion about physicians because we've all been patients. Many of us have also worked with physicians and have a variety of experiences to report about their attitudes toward nonphysician health professionals. Physicians, or medical doctors, hold the Doctor of Medicine (MD) or Doctor of Osteopathic Medicine (DO) degree. They are licensed to practice medicine in all states and territories. Medical school graduation is only the beginning of a long period of clinical education and training, ranging from residencies of perhaps two to five or more years, depending upon the area of specialization. Written examinations are required for licensure, as well as board certification in a specialty area (e.g., neurology, pediatrics, psychiatry, otolaryngology).

The medical profession might be called the profession in transition. Forces in the health-care system are rapidly changing the ways physicians practice. The sanctity and exclusivity of the doctor-patient relationship are lessening as employers increasingly require that employees obtain second opinions for elective surgery and approval for hospital admissions. The entire hospital stay is monitored for "medical necessity." Days in a hospital that an insurance company's nurse reviewer finds unneccessary may not be covered. For high-cost illnesses and injuries case managers (employed by insurance companies and consulting firms) monitor and approve every service and procedure that a patient receives. As a result, often physicians must consult with and receive authorization for patient-care services from a growing variety of management personnel.

Komaroff (1985) contends that traditional fee-for-service physician solo practices are rapidly dying. Instead, physicians are moving into large group practices and networks as well as affiliating with alternative delivery systems such as HMOs and PPOs. Of the nation's 500,000 physicians, more than 85,000 currently practice in HMOs and PPOs. It has also been estimated that 50% of all physicians will be salaried employees of health systems by 1990.

Doctors have been the traditional directors of patient care. Used to giving orders, they are willing to accept final responsibility for their patients, as well as the liability for errors in patient care. They are beginning to recognize, however, that nonphysician health-care professionals also have expertise, but the process of relinquishing some authority to allied health professionals is not without frustrations and controversies. At the same time nonphysician health professionals are declaring themselves independent, the health-care system is moving away from that mode, even for physicians. Licensure laws notwithstanding, many companies continue to require that physicians refer, recommend, or order the services of allied health professionals. The Medicare program requires that physicians verify the need for allied health services, and the program must periodically recertify that services are "medically necessary."

Despite arguments to the contrary, physicians are still the central figures in health care. Most people access the health-care system through their physicians. Consequently, physicians are a valuable referral source. We can build bridges with them by cultivating our professional relationships through formal and informal education about communication disorders and speech-language pathology and audiology services and by attempting to meet their needs better. Physicians can also be recipients of referrals from speech-language pathologists and audiologists. In today's evolving health-care system, the door is open for further collaboration and cooperation between physicians and other health-care professionals.

Nurses

Nursing isn't what it used to be—it's a lot more! Not so long ago, most registered nurses (RNs) received their training in two-year hospital-based nursing education programs. They were regarded primarily as doctor's helpers and were not permitted to make many decisions themselves. Today, nurses are assuming greater authority and responsibility as health-care professionals, and they are likely to hold the Bachelor of Science in Nursing (BSN) or Master of Science in Nursing (MSN) degree. A few states now require the baccalaureate degree to qualify for RN licensure. Some nurse executives and most professors of nursing and researchers hold the Doctor of Philosophy (PhD) degree.

As health care has become more complex, nurses, like other health-care practitioners, are specializing in certain areas of practice (e.g., pediatrics, gerontology, surgery, emergency and trauma, rehabilitation) and are attempting to increase their visibility as primary health-care providers. In addition to academic degree programs, there are a number of advanced training programs. For example, nurse practitioners (NP) are licensed RNs who have prepared themselves for an expanded role in the delivery of health-care services by completing a one-year formal academic program leading to certification. The Association of Rehabilitation Nurses (ARN) awards the designation Certified Registered Rehabilitation Nurse (CRRN) to individuals who have completed at least two years of professional rehabilitation nursing experience, have passed a written examination, and have been recommended by colleagues. After five years, recertification is attained by reexamination, publishing in professional journals, or proof of continuing education. The titles *nurse clinician, clinical coordinator,* and *clinical nurse specialist* are usually held by nurses who hold master's degrees, have a number of years of clinical experience, and have participated in advanced continuing education opportunities.

Nurses work in virtually all settings in which health-care services are offered: hospitals, clinics, health maintenance organizations, health departments, physicians' offices, business and industry, the military, and schools. In some cases, nurses have private practices (e.g., nurse-midwives). Although direct reimbursement for nursing services is currently the exception, it is a growing trend. In addition to providing patient care, nurses have increasing opportunities in management and administration. Utilization review and quality assurance activities in hospitals and other settings are largely conducted by nurses. Insurance companies, third-party administrators, and consulting firms hire predominantly nurses for claims review, case management, and medical auditing positions.

Speech-language pathologists who work in health care will have frequent contact with the nursing staff, especially on neurology, rehabilitation, trauma, and pediatric units. Nurses are excellent information and referral sources, as well as integral members of the patient-care team. The nurse can be a liaison to physicians, other health professionals, and the patient's family. She or he can also extend SLP activities throughout the patient's inpatient stay and serve as an advocate for postdischarge SLP services.

To obtain information about the scope of nursing practice as it pertains to rehabilitation nursing, we consulted the 1987 *Accreditation Manual for Hospitals* (*AMH*), published by the Joint Commission on Accreditation of Hospitals. According to the *AMH*, the goal of rehabilitation nursing is to provide for the prevention of complications of physical disability, the restoration of optimal functioning, and adaptation to an altered life-style through the use of the nursing process. These processes include assessments of the patient's self-care skills; interpersonal relations; cognitive functioning; sleep and rest patterns; adaptive mechanisms and patterns for managing stress; and nutrition, hydration, appetite, and dietary habits. Rehabilitation nursing interventions encompass physical and psychosocial care, reinforcement of the interdisciplinary treatment plan, evaluation of the effectiveness of nursing interventions, health maintenance, and discharge teaching.

Established in 1896, the American Nurses Association (ANA) represents the interests of America's registered nurses. This professional association has about 200,000 members, with 53 state and territorial organizations and 900 district associations of nurses. The ANA maintains programs for specialty certification in 17 areas of nursing practice; accredits continuing education programs in nursing; and sets standards for nursing practice, education, and credentialing, among many other activities. In its long-range plan the ANA has established goals to expand the scientific and research base for nursing practice, strengthen the educational and credentialing system for nursing, restructure the organizational arrangements for delivery of nursing services, and develop comprehensive payment systems for financing nursing services.

Physical Therapists

Physical therapists plan, organize, conduct, and evaluate rehabilitation programs for the care of individuals whose ability to function is impaired or threatened by illness, injury, or birth defects. Focusing upon individuals who present disorders related to musculoskeletal, neurological, pulmonary, and cardiovascular systems, physical therapists concentrate on the objectives of preventing disability and pain, restoring function and relieving pain, promoting healing, and facilitating adaptation to permanent disability. Assessment and treatment activities conducted by physical therapists are summarized in Figure 6.1.

About 40% of physical therapists work in hospitals, but the profession is rapidly expanding to many other settings. Physical therapists also provide services in home-care agencies, schools, outpatient clinics, long-term-care facilities and hospices, academic institutions, business and industry, and private offices. Private practice is a growing trend in the field. In industry, physical therapists conduct programs related to health awareness, safety education, and injury management. They also evaluate the safety of a company's work facilities as well as conduct comprehensive functional assessments that consider individual employees' capabilities and limitations in doing certain types of work.

FIGURE 6.1
Physical Therapy Assessment and Treatment Activities

Physical Therapy Assessments
- Joint range of motion and mobility
- Skeletal muscle strength
- Reflexes and muscle tonus
- Posture and gait
- Pulmonary function
- Sensory perception and sensory/motor nerve conduction
- Sensorimotor performance
- Orthotic/prosthetic fit and function

Physical Therapy Interventions
- Transfer skills
- Positioning, seating, and postural control
- Joint-mobilization and range-of-motion exercises
- Training in use of orthotic, prosthetic, and other adaptive and assistive devices
- Therapeutic exercises for strengthening muscular, respiratory, and cardiovascular systems
- Ambulation training and mobility training in activities of daily living
- Skin-care management
- Therapeutic massage and relaxation training
- Biofeedback
- Modalities
    Ultrasound
    Traction
    Diathermy
    Electrotherapy
    Cryotherapy
    Hydrotherapy

The educational credentials currently required to practice physical therapy (PT) are obtained in one of three ways: (1) a bachelor's degree in physical therapy, (2) a certificate in physical therapy for those persons who have a bachelor's degree in a related field, or (3) a graduate degree in physical therapy. The profession is moving toward graduate-level preparation for entry into the field. Physical therapists are licensed in all 50 states, the District of Columbia, the Virgin Islands, and Puerto Rico. Thirteen states permit direct access to physical therapy; that is, no medical prescription or referral is required for patients to receive physical therapy treatment. Thirty-six states permit PT evaluations without physician referral. The American Board of Physical Therapy Specialties recognizes the following areas of expertise: neurologic, cardiopulmonary, clinical electrophysiology, orthopedics, pediatrics, and sports medicine.

The American Physical Therapy Association (APTA) is the national professional association that represents more than 45,000 physical therapists and physical therapy assistants (health technicians who work under the direction and supervision of a physical therapist). APTA's goals are to increase understanding of the physical therapist's role in the health-care system and to improve physical therapy education, practice, and research in order to meet the physical therapy needs of all citizens. APTA publishes the journal *Physical Therapy* as well as a number of other periodicals.

Physical therapists and speech-language pathologists may interact in several ways in both health-care and educational settings. Their relationship may include mutual referrals, consultation, collaboration, and even business partnership. Physical therapists and speech-language pathologists can help each other carry out patient treatment goals. In addition to exchanging information during case staffings or team meetings, physical therapists and speech-language pathologists may directly participate in the other's therapy sessions. For example, the speech-language pathologist may be present during PT treatment sessions to facilitate communication between the physical therapist and his or her patient, or to instruct the patient or physical therapist in specific communication strategies. The physical therapist can then reinforce SLP treatment goals during PT sessions, as well as communicate more effectively with the patient. Conversely, the physical therapist may teach the speech-language pathologist how to help patients accomplish transfers or walk with minimal assistance, or how to reposition patients in their wheelchairs. In addition, the speech-language pathologist may extend and generalize PT activities during SLP sessions by creating opportunities for the patient to practice physical activities during communication interactions.

Speech-language pathologists and physical therapists can help sensitize each other to patient behaviors that may indicate the need for SLP/A or PT evaluations. Both professionals benefit from mutual inservice education opportunities, whether the work setting is a hospital, an educational institution, or a private practice. Private practitioners in SLP and PT may want to encourage networking to generate referrals and heighten interprofessional cooperation and continuity of patient care. It should be noted here that in some states the speech-language pathologist must first contact the patient's physician in order to secure a referral to a physical therapist for an evaluation. All but 13 states require physician referral for PT treatment.

Finally, the Medicare rehabilitation agency (RA) provider type provides one way in which physical therapists and speech-language pathologists may become business partners as well as collaborators in their overall goal of providing quality rehabilitation services to their patients. Rehabilitation agencies may be established by a speech-language pathologist or a physical therapist (or both). Social or vocational adjustment services must also be offered as needed for a patient's rehabilitation program. More information about rehabilitation agencies is found in chapter 7.

Occupational Therapists

Occupational therapy is the art and science of directing human participation in selected tasks to restore, reinforce, and enhance performance; to facilitate learning of those skills and functions essential for adaptation and productivity; to diminish or correct pathology; and to promote and maintain health. The term *occupation* refers to goal-directed use of time, energy, interest, and attention to maintain satisfactory performance of the essential activities of daily living. Services are provided to people whose lives have been threatened or disrupted by physical injury or illness, developmental problems, the aging process, and social/psychological difficulties.

Occupational therapists assess the client's functional abilities related to the following areas: occupational performance (work, self-care, leisure); performance components (sensorimotor, cognitive, psychosocial); and therapeutic adaptations and prevention. According to the American Occupational Therapy Association (1979), *treatment* refers to "the use of specific activities or methods to develop, improve, and/or restore the performance of necessary functions; compensate for dysfunction; and/or minimize debilitation; and the planning for and documenting of treatment performance." The scope of occupational therapy practice is outlined in Figure 6.2.

The minimum requirement for entry into the field of occupational therapy includes a baccalaureate degree with a major in occupational therapy, with a year-long internship as part of the education and training process. The title *Occupational Therapist, Registered* (OTR) is awarded to individuals who have met specified education and training requirements and who have passed a national registration examination. OTs are licensed in 34 states, and 2 states have trademark laws for the use of the title. The Master of Occupational Therapy (MOT) is the entry-level degree for persons who have earned bachelor's degrees in other fields. OTs may also earn master's and doctoral degrees in occupational therapy or related fields. Currently, the trend is toward earning advanced degrees in business or technology.

The American Occupational Therapy Association (AOTA) represents approximately 32,400 OTRs and 7,750 Certified Occupational Therapy Assistants (COTA) in the United States. COTAs work under the direction and supervision

FIGURE 6.2
Scope of Occupational Therapy Practice

Independent Living/Daily Living Skills
  Physical Daily Living Skills
    Grooming and Hygiene
    Feeding/Eating
    Dressing
    Functional Mobility
    Functional Communication
    Object Manipulation
  Psychological/Emotional Daily Living Skills
    Self-concept/Self-identity
    Situational Coping
    Community Involvement
  Work
    Homemaking
    Child Care/Parenting
    Employment Preparation
  Play/Leisure
Sensorimotor Components
  Neuromuscular
    Reflex Integration
    Range of Motion
    Gross and Fine Coordination
    Strength and Endurance
  Sensory Integration
    Sensory Awareness
    Visual-Spatial Awareness
    Body Integration

Cognitive Components
  Orientation
  Conceptualization/Comprehension
    Concentration
    Attention Span
    Memory
  Cognitive Integration
    Generalization
    Problem Solving
Psychosocial Components
  Self-management
    Self-expression
    Self-control
  Dyadic Interaction
  Group Interaction
Therapeutic Adaptations
  Orthotics
  Prosthetics
  Assistive/Adaptive Equipments
Prevention
  Energy Conservation
  Joint Protection/Body Mechanics
  Positioning
  Coordination of Daily Living Activities

NOTE: Based on information from *Uniform Terminology for Reporting Occupational Therapy Services* by American Occupational Therapy Association, March 1979, by Rockville, MD: AOTA.

of registered occupational therapists. Most assistants have associate degrees, but they may also earn certificates in occupational therapy. OTs work in hospitals, rehabilitation centers, sheltered workshops, universities, long-term-care facilities, industry, schools, home-care agencies, and private practice. About 6% of the private practitioners have their own offices; 20% are independent contractors.

Numerous opportunities exist in health-care and education settings for speech-language pathologists and occupational therapists to collaborate and consult, for example, with persons having brain injury, stroke, neurogenic and neuromuscular diseases, and developmental and learning disabilities. Unfortunately, practitioners have also encountered problems with overlap and duplication of services, because occupational therapists and speech-language pathologists have areas of common interest. In response to these concerns, ASHA has established an ad hoc committee with the American Occupational Therapy Association. Its charge is to develop mutual understanding and definition of roles of practice with reference to the evaluation and treatment of dysphagia, cognitive impairments, and severely handicapped nonspeaking children and adults. Each association will develop information packets for their respective memberships detailing the agreed-upon areas of practice and guidelines for interprofessional cooperation and consultation.

Psychologists

Psychology is the science of behavior; the field of psychology focuses on the understanding of behavior and the environmental conditions that may precipitate behavior. Psychologists are concerned with both individual and group behavior as well as community and societal problems. Areas of specialization within the practice of psychology are numerous:

clinical	forensic
cognitive	general
community	health
comparative	industrial and organizational
consulting	neuropsychology
counseling	personality
educational	psychometric/quantitative
engineering	rehabilitation
environmental	school
experimental	social

Consequently, practice settings vary widely. According to a census conducted by Stapp, Tucker, and VandenBos (1985), primary employment settings for psychologists, in descending order, are academic, independent practice, hospitals and clinics, business and government, other human services, and education. All 50 states and the District of Columbia have licensure laws for the independent practice of psychology. Most states require the doctoral degree (PhD, EdD, or PsyD) and two years of supervised experience for licensure.

Speech-language pathologists work with clinical psychologists, neuropsychologists, rehabilitation psychologists, or health psychologists in health-care settings. Clinical psychologists assess and treat a broad range of mental and emotional disorders. Some may focus their interests on a specific population, such as children or elderly persons, or on certain diagnoses (e.g., eating disorders, depression, or psychoses).

Neuropsychologists study the relation of brain structure to function and the chemical and physical changes associated with emotional/mental states. They also diagnose behavioral disturbances related to suspected dysfunction of the

central nervous system. In addition, neuropsychologists treat cognitive disturbances through methods generically called "cognitive retraining." Speech-language pathologists also participate in the evaluation and treatment of cognitively
based communication disorders. The relationship between the work of neuropsychologists and speech-language pathologists in the treatment of cognitive
disorders is discussed in the ASHA (1987a) report "The Role of Speech-Language
Pathologists in the Habilitation and Rehabilitation of Cognitively-Impaired
Individuals."

Rehabilitation psychologists work with physically and mentally disabled
individuals who require assistance in adjusting to their disabilities and in overcoming barriers to achieving functional independence. Rehabilitation psychologists usually work in medical rehabilitation centers, universities, and private
practice. They also serve as consultants to vocational rehabilitation agencies.

Health psychology is a new specialty within the field. These psychologists
are concerned with the contributions of psychology to health-promotion and
health-maintenance programs, as well as the prevention of illness and disease.
Health psychologists may work in medical centers, health maintenance organizations, industry, public health agencies, and private practice.

In educational settings speech-language pathologists often work with school
psychologists. These professionals assess and monitor the intellectual, social, and
emotional development of children. They also plan and conduct intervention
programs for individual children as well as provide consultation to classroom
teachers and other professionals on learning techniques, behavior management,
and other aspects of the overall learning environment. School psychologists and
speech-language pathologists serve together on multidisciplinary teams that
assess children suspected of having language-learning disabilities or other handicaps. With other members of the team they determine appropriate educational
placements and individualized programs for children who are diagnosed as
having language-learning disorders. For more information about the roles of
speech-language pathologists and school psychologists in evaluating and treating
language-learning disorders, see ASHA (1987b).

In contrast to other psychology specialists about 70% of school psychologists
hold nondoctoral degrees (i.e., master's or specialist). Of the nation's 20,000
school psychologists, about 9,500 are represented by the National Association of
School Psychologists (NASP). Those who are members of Division 16 of the
American Psychological Association must hold doctoral degrees.

The American Psychological Association (APA) is the professional society
organized to advance psychology as a science and to promote the public welfare.
It has more than 62,000 members, who belong to 1 or more of 42 divisions. Most
divisions or interest areas publish a journal or newsletter, and the APA publishes
24 psychological journals.

Social Workers

Social work seeks to help individuals, groups, and communities reach the highest
possible degree of social, mental, and physical well-being. Social work interven-

tions are implemented with consideration of the dynamic interplay among social, economic, and psychological factors that influence human lives. The National Association of Social Workers has referred to social work as "the profession in the middle."

In general, the goal of social work is to reconcile the well-being of individuals with the welfare of the society in which they live. Social workers help clients alter their environment as well as the ways they interact in family and society. Social work is based on the belief that people are capable of changing attitudes and behaviors and that the strategies people need to change as they desire can be communicated and learned.

Traditionally, the major divisions within social work practice have distinguished between change efforts directed at macrosystems—such as organizations and communities—and those aimed at microsystems—such as individuals, families, and small groups. Both direct- and indirect-intervention strategies are used. Two examples of indirect interventions are government agency work advocacy and referral consultations. Direct-service examples include client counseling sessions, in-home child-welfare casework, and assistance to low-income families through financial planning activities. There are 10 primary social work specialties: child welfare, public welfare, drug and alcohol abuse; mental health; health care; family service; developmental disabilities; industry, business, and labor; schools and youth; and services to the aged. About one third of social workers work in health-care settings.

Health-care or medical social workers are often the primary advocates for patients' rights. They may coordinate communication between the patient-care team and the patient's family. Medical social workers may also specialize in assisting patients in specific hospital units such as oncology, trauma, neonatology, or rehabilitation. The social work department usually also directs or coordinates discharge-planning activities. As length of stay in acute-care facilities decreases, discharge planning is of primary importance in placing patients in appropriate postacute settings. Social workers may be able to help speech-language pathologists assure continuity of speech-language-hearing services by helping to arrange for provision of the services in postdischarge settings such as long-term-care facilities and home-care agencies.

Social workers who provide services to pupils in school systems contribute a knowledge of and sensitivity to the range of influences that affect the teaching and learning process. The social worker is concerned with such needs and problems of students as absenteeism and truancy, delinquency, substance abuse, interpersonal conflicts, teenage pregnancy, economic deprivation, domestic violence, child abuse, divorce, effects of unemployment on the family, inadequate health care, and suicidal and self-destructive behavior. School social workers also have an essential role in providing services to handicapped students. A social assessment is mandated by the Education for All Handicapped Children Act (PL 94–142).

Social work interventions are related to learning opportunities, academic achievement, interpersonal functioning, and need for change in the student's school and home environment. The focus of social work in the school setting is on working with the intra- and interpersonal and social systems that may contribute to or alleviate a student's identified problems.

Both direct and indirect methods are used to accomplish the goals of school social work. Some examples are

- Outreach and liason between school, home, and community;
- Planning and evaluation of preventive and developmental student services;
- Staff development and consultation;
- Individual, group, and family counseling.

School social workers and speech-language pathologists may find many opportunities for mutual referrals and consultations. During the course of an interview with a child about a problem at home or in school, the social worker may suspect that the child has a language problem and then refer the student for a speech-language evaluation. The speech-language pathologist is often the only professional, besides the classroom teacher, with whom a student has regular contact. Therefore, the SLP should be attuned to children's statements and behaviors that may signal the need for a referral to the social worker. In some cases it may be appropriate for the school social worker and speech-language pathologist to make a joint home visit to assess a student's home environment and family communication patterns. This type of partnership, which requires mutual education, support, and cooperation, can be very rewarding for the speech-language pathologist, the social worker, and the students and families served.

The preferred credential for social work practice is the Master of Social Work degree (MSW), which includes 900 hours of supervised internship experiences. Social workers are certified by their national professional association and licensed in 36 states. The highest credential of social work practice is the Academy of Certified Social Workers (ACSW). This designation is earned by meeting the following requirements: (1) membership in the National Association of Social Workers; (2) attainment of the MSW degree; (3) completion of two years of full-time social work experience under the supervision of a holder of the ACSW; and (4) passing of a national examination. Social workers may also earn doctoral degrees (Doctors of Philosophy or Doctor of Social Work).

The National Association of Social Workers (NASW), with 90,000 members and 55 chapters, is the largest association of professional social workers in the world. NASW's primary functions include encouraging professional development, establishing standards of practice, and advancing responsible national social policies. NASW is committed to the eradication of poverty and racism from our society.

Educators

Educators are people who specialize in helping others learn. They use certain techniques or methods to facilitate the process of gathering, processing, and understanding information. These professionals work with all age groups and in diverse employment settings, some of which include preschools, day-care centers, elementary and secondary schools, colleges and universities, public and private agencies, business and industry, health-care facilities, and private practice. Titles may vary from director of medical education to continuing education coordinator to the more generic designations of professor, learning disabilities specialist, or classroom teacher.

Speech-language pathologists may work with many educators, but generally they interact with public and private school teachers more often than with other educators. Classroom teachers are central figures in public education and should be regarded as integral members of multidisciplinary teams in schools. A child's teacher can contribute valuable information about his or her physical, emotional, academic, and social behaviors as well as assist other professionals in implementing goals and objectives. As the focus of special education shifts from compartmentalized to integrated services for handicapped children, the classroom teacher is increasingly called upon to coordinate and carry out classroom generalization, or mainstreaming activities as recommended by the specialists who are directing the student's Individual Education Plan (IEP). Additionally, innovative speech-language pathology service delivery models in education such as the indirect or consultation model and in-class treatment approaches require the collaboration and cooperation of the classroom teacher and speech-language pathologist to achieve the desired objectives. It is important to remember that the classroom teacher is the primary referral source for speech-language caseloads and is also a valuable liaison to parents, administrators, other professionals, and students.

The minimum requirement for state provisional certification as a regular classroom teacher is the bachelor's degree. Permanent certification is earned by successful completion of postbaccalaureate academic credits and a specified number of years of teaching experience. Many elementary and secondary school teachers earn master's degrees, and in some school districts, many also have specialist and doctoral degrees. Additional certification is required for educators who provide special education services (for example, for students with learning disabilities or those who are mentally, emotionally, or physically impaired). In many states, speech-language pathologists who work in schools must also be certified teachers.

The National Education Association (NEA) and the American Federation of Teachers (AFT) represent the interests of the majority of the nation's 2.1 million teachers. The NEA has approximately 1.5 million members, and the AFT has 450,000 members. Representing primarily urban educators, the AFT has promoted educational reform and research, whereas the NEA has focused its efforts in suburban and rural areas. The NEA is known as a very active organization politically, and it strongly advocates the professionalization of teaching.

THE TEAM CONCEPT

The team approach to health care is an outgrowth of the post–World War II knowledge explosion. As medicine became more complex, the numbers and types of health personnel also grew. Allied health professionals were needed to assist physicians, the primary health caregivers. The label *allied health* was initially conceived as an umbrella term for all workers who participated in the delivery of health care in a supplemental or supporting relationship to physicians. This definition was based upon a hierarchical structure in which allied health personnel took orders from physicians and had very little autonomy.

As the new fields developed, each allied health occupation or profession sought to establish its own identity and area of expertise. Accreditation, certification, registration, and licensure laws defined specific scopes of practice. Division of labor in the overall health-care process became highly specialized. According to Pellegrino (1977), the result was "a confusing array of technical and professional personnel working in compartmentalized tasks, often closely overlapping each other in some facet of their work and frequently out of communication with each other about the patient whom they presumably both serve" (p. 27). Team approaches were offered as the answer to the fragmentation of patient care. Today, the patient-care team is an evolving and dynamic concept with plenty of room for refinement.

What exactly is a team? Lowe (1978) defines it as "a group of people, each of whom possesses particular expertise; each of whom is responsible for making decisions; who together hold a common purpose; who meet together to communicate, collaborate, and consolidate knowledge from which plans are made, actions determined and future decisions influenced" (p. 324). *Webster's Unabridged Dictionary* describes teamwork as "joint action by a group of people, in which each person subordinates his individual interests and opinions to the unity and efficiency of the group." The purpose and composition of teams vary with the needs of patients, team members, organizations, and institutions. Teams may always be regarded as a pool of human resources gathered to solve problems cooperatively. The degree to which team members work together depends upon the team's organizational model. Three types are discussed in the next sections: multidisciplinary, interdisciplinary, and transdisciplinary teams.

Multidisciplinary and Interdisciplinary Approaches to Patient Care

When is a team a team? The terms *multidisciplinary* and *interdisciplinary* are often used interchangeably, but they mean different things to different people. According to Clark (1979), the key feature distinguishing between the two models is the degree of collaboration and interdependence required among team members. If we strictly adhere to our definitions of *team*, there is some question whether multidisciplinary teams are teams at all. Watkins (1983) maintains that "multidisciplinary refers to individuals from several disciplines whose efforts are discipline-oriented and though focused on a common purpose and goal, a group effort is not required" (p. 439). For example, a multidisciplinary team patient assessment in one hospital may mean nothing more than a group of health professionals conducting separate evaluations and reporting results during a meeting or contributing reports to the medical record. Treatment sessions are conducted by individual departments, and there may not be subsequent meetings to exchange information and recommendations for continued patient care.

We know of one hospital in which a quasi-team approach was followed. Representatives were sent by various departments to weekly lunch-hour meetings in which individual patients who were receiving rehabilitation services were discussed. Nursing personnel coordinated the meetings and recorded information presented for later discussion with the patient's physician. Physicians never actually attended the meetings; the hospital administration never officially recognized the team; rehabilitation personnel met on their lunch hour because time for interprofessional meetings was not designated in their schedules. Although not the best of situations, the quasi-team at least established interprofessional and interdepartmental communication and may have improved patient care.

The multidisciplinary team approach has received considerable support in the public sector. Federal laws and regulations require that a team approach be used in evaluating and treating persons who participate in certain governmental programs. The Education for All Handicapped Children Act (PL 94-142) mandates that initial assessment of students suspected of having a handicap be made by "a multidisciplinary team or group of persons, including at least one teacher or other specialist with knowledge in the area of suspected disability" (34 CFR 300.532). Parents must also be included in educational planning and placement. The team requirement under PL 94-142 includes assessment, development of the Individualized Education Plan (IEP), yearly IEP review, and reevaluation of the child every three years, or more frequently if conditions warrant or a child's parent or teacher requests an evaluation. The degree to which education professionals maintain contact during implementation of the IEP (the school year), however, is a matter of staff discretion.

Interdisciplinary team approaches involve high levels of coordination and integration of services, but they are also subject to greater potential for interprofessional conflicts as a result of the collaboration required. Interdisciplinary teams are composed of representatives of different professions, but their activities are directed toward group-defined goals according to individual patient needs. Melvin (1980) asserts that "this effort requires the skills necessary for effective group interaction and the knowledge of how to transfer integrated group activities into a result which is greater than the simple sum of the activities of each individual discipline" (p. 380). Team members recognize their interdependence and organize their work so that services are integrated. This process may be divided into phases, as outlined in Figure 6.3. Each phase requires negotiation and cooperation among team members. During Phase I, data collection, the team delineates the roles and responsibilities of each professional for a particular patient's care. These roles vary depending upon the patient's needs and the practitioners' expertise and interests. Information needs of team participants are also identified so that accurate patient evaluations can be conducted. In Phase II the team members analyze and coordinate the information gathered; diagnoses are offered in preparation for treatment planning in Phase III. The intervention process, Phase IV, may be very creative in the interdisciplinary model. For

FIGURE 6.3
Phases of Interdisciplinary Functioning

I. Data Collection

Identification of roles, responsibilities, team-member information needs.

II. Data Assessment

Interpretation and integration of information; diagnoses made based upon contributions of each professional.

III. Decision Making

Options evaluated; treatment plans developed; treatment tasks assigned to team members for implementation by process of negotiation and consultation.

IV. Treatment

Intervention services delivered.

V. Evaluation

Treatment process and patient outcomes evaluated; individual and collective performance of team appraised.

example, in one comprehensive medical rehabilitation center, the speech-language pathologist and occupational therapist conduct a joint treatment session for a CVA patient while the rehabilitation psychologist observes the session. Later, the three professionals discuss the session and modify some activities for the next day. That same day, the speech-language pathologist meets with the patient and his or her vocational counselor to design functional activities to facilitate the patient's return to work. In Phase V the team assesses individual and collective team efforts. Monitoring and evaluation of treatment effectiveness and efficiency, as well as team communication and management, are ongoing processes.

The interdisciplinary approach seems to coordinate patient care better, but there is little empirical evidence that such teams effect qualitative improvements in service delivery per se or that the system is less costly than nonteam patient care. In fact, the implementation of team approaches may require more personnel, increased staff training, modification or expansion of facilities, and increased consultation and patient-contact time. Additionally, team organization and practice patterns may not be compatible with some legal, quasi-legal, institutional, and educational requirements for professional practices.

Requirements for professional education, certification, and program accreditation sometimes present barriers to successful implementation of team approaches. Practitioners who are completing coursework and clinical practicum experiences to meet minimum professional standards may devote very little time to working with students or interacting with other professionals, or to developing problem-solving, management, and group-process skills necessary for building viable health teams. Without a common knowledge base, one professional may define his or her role in a way that is incongruent with the perceptions of others. Resistance to sharing information, defensiveness and turf protection, and duplication of services result from a lack of information and poor communication among professionals. Most practitioners have been trained to perform highly specialized and independent services. As members of a health team, however, professionals must be willing to relinquish a certain amount of autonomy in order to participate in a collaborative, interdependent effort.

Changing service delivery models demand that professionals seek new ways of working together. This challenge is very evident for speech-language pathologists who work in schools. Consultation models require high levels of collaboration between speech-language pathologists, other special educators, and classroom teachers, as well as the support of administrators. Suggestions for consultation approaches have been presented by Pickering (1981); Frassinelli, Superior, and Meyers (1983); and the American Speech-Language-Hearing Association (1984). As speech-language pathologists expand their roles in schools to include evaluation of teachers and curriculum language as well as classroom communication patterns (see Nelson, 1984, 1985; and Simon, 1985), the need for skillful interprofessional interaction increases. Tomes and Sanger (1986) surveyed the attitudes of other team members toward speech-language pathology services in public schools. Results suggested that educators generally had positive attitudes toward these services but were sometimes confused about the SLP's role within the team. Some respondents also questioned the feasibility of management suggestions provided to classroom teachers by speech-language pathologists. Tomes and Sanger recommended that SLPs increase contact with other school professionals by soliciting their suggestions for treatment plans and inservice programs, and by initiating other types of formal and informal interactions.

There is no single model for describing the expectations and interactions of team members. Each group of professionals brings unique experiences, knowledge, expertise, and personalities to the team. In addition, the organization and activities of the team may be governed or influenced by the policies of facility or program administrators. A speech-language pathologist in one setting may frequently serve as team leader, whereas in another facility the speech-language pathologist may struggle to establish an appropriate and satisfying role within the team structure.

A team is composed of human beings. Therefore, the team can experience a wide range of interactions and effects. The work of the team may be synergistic or fragmented; and its impact on patient care may be positive, neutral, or negative. The members must strive to work together on both technical and personal levels. Expertise in one's own profession is only part of the game. Successful team members also understand the skills and contributions of other professionals, have group-process and interpersonal communication skills, and develop collegial leadership styles. Finally, collaboration, cooperation, and compromise might be called the "three Cs" of a successful team approach. These attributes are particularly important in the third type of team model to be discussed here—the transdisciplinary approach to patient care.

Transdisciplinary Teams and Multiskilled Health Practitioners

The transdisciplinary, or integrative, model is perhaps the most innovative, yet controversial, patient-care team approach. Introduced by Hutchinson in 1974, the term *transdisciplinary* was used to describe the organizational model of some of the United Cerebral Palsy Collaborative Infant Programs in which a group of professionals provided consultation and support for one primary implementor (McCormick & Lee, 1979). Figure 6.4 contains a diagram of the transdisciplinary service system. Each team member is responsible for an initial patient assessment as well as a treatment plan. The implementation of treatment objectives is usually assigned to the team member whose expertise corresponds to the patient's primary presenting problem. Other team members provide ongoing consultation and assistance to the implementor. As McCormick and Lee point out, transdisciplinary approaches can "broaden the sphere of influence" (p. 588) for individual professionals, because more patients can be served than would be possible if each professional delivered separate services in individual treatment sessions.

Watkins (1984) described the following outpatient treatment scenario, based upon the transdisciplinary model:

> Mrs. Smith is a middle-aged woman who is recovering from a stroke, has aphasia, lives alone, and will return to work. Due to a limited inpatient stay, she was unable to complete some of the objectives of her treatment plan, including adaptive homemaking skills, hand dexterity, and increasing endurance in ambulation. Her outpatient therapy program was planned prior to discharge by all appropriate members of the rehabilitation team. Her primary outpatient therapist will be an occupational therapist. The OT will facilitate Mrs. Smith's hand dexterity, carry-over speech-language activities, including writing, and incorporate ambulation endurance goals into work-related activities as well as self-care and home maintenance.

In a second scenario described by Watkins (1984), the speech-language pathologist will implement team goals:

> Mr. Jones is a stroke patient who is a business executive. Due to partial paralysis and obesity, Mr. Jones will not be a functional ambulator and will use a wheelchair. His primary residual deficits are in high-level language skills. The speech-language pathologist will consult with the vocational counselor and the patient's employer in preparation for Mr. Jones's return to work, and will also continue activities to improve fine motor coordination.

Both examples illustrate the need for rehabilitation professionals who can highly integrate services to meet individual patients' needs. Cross-training and cross-utilization are mandatory. Currently, the transdisciplinary model is not widely used, but there is growing support for this type of patient care.

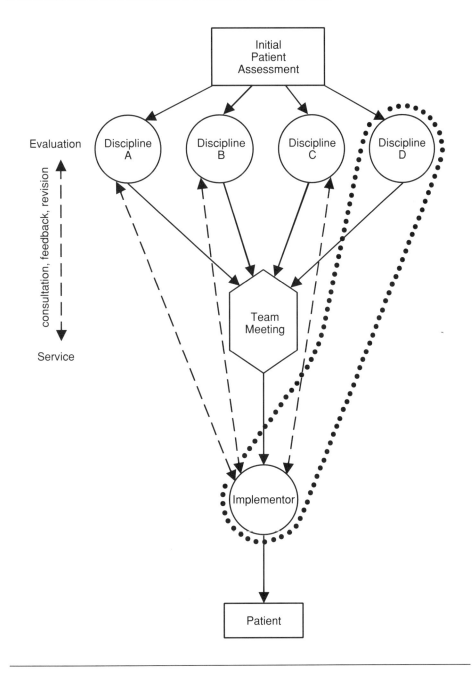

FIGURE 6.4

Transdisciplinary Service System

NOTE: Adapted from ''Public Law 94–142: Mandated Partnerships'' by L. McCormick and C. Lee, 1979, *American Journal of Occupational Therapy, 33*(9), Figure 1. Copyright 1979 by the American Occupational Therapy Association, Inc. Reprinted with permission.

During the past 15 years, the focus of health professionals has become highly specialized. Hospitals and other health-care programs have hired numerous clinicians, technicians, and technologists to perform distinct functions. Many analysts believe that the health-care system has become too cumbersome and that services are fragmented and duplicative. Since the early 1980s, the health-care system has stressed the importance of cost containment and establishment of alternative service delivery systems. These trends favor a restructuring of the health-care workforce to develop more efficient and cost-effective ways to utilize health-care personnel.

Traditionally, medical rehabilitation services have been labor intensive. England (1986) observed that the large rehabilitation team is probably no longer practical as more services move to the outpatient setting. He predicts that new kinds of rehabilitation professionals will emerge—supertherapists—whose skills cross current disciplinary boundaries. *Supertherapist* is one of several terms used to describe what may be the health-care professional of the future: the multiskilled, skill-enhanced, or expanded-skill health-care practitioner. According to Blayney (1986), the intent behind the multicompetency movement "is not to encroach on the legitimate realms of other allied health or nursing personnel, but to organize the work environment so that more tasks can be performed without the awkward assignment of a variety of over-specialized people. Hospitals, HMOs, and others in health care delivery can no longer afford the luxury of underemployed staff" (p. 277).

Multicompetency training is provided in both hospitals and colleges or universities. Thus far, the majority of programs have targeted clinical technical occupations. For example, the multiple competency clinical technician (MCCT) program at the University of Alabama's School of Community and Allied Health trains technicians in medical assisting with additional instruction in radiography and medical laboratory technology. Southern Illinois University offers a "skill enhancement" program in which students, many of whom are already certified in one specialty, return to school to extend their knowledge and skills in related areas. According to administrators, these programs are not necessarily designed to prepare students for dual licensure or certification but to add certain competencies to the technician's repertoire (Lugenbeel, 1986; Morgan, 1986). New multicompetency programs are developing rapidly and are beginning to extend to professional areas such as nursing and physical and occupational therapies. Bamberg and Blayney (1984) reported in their survey that physical and occupational therapists felt the need for additional training in areas such as vocational evaluation, rehabilitation counseling, social work, psychology, and special education as well as each other's area of expertise. Physical therapists also wanted to know more about prosthetics, orthotics, and emergency room procedures, and OTs desired more skills in art and recreation therapies.

As the multiskilled-practitioner movement grows, more questions will be raised about the implications for professional practice in view of current licensure laws and accreditation and certification standards. Where does skill enhancement end and violation of licensure laws begin? Will quality of patient care suffer as so-called generalist practitioners try to do some of the work of three other professionals? Will a multicompetent nurse be held liable for errors in patient care if she or he performs within the scope of practice of a licensed physical therapist or speech-language pathologist? Larkins (1987) observed that there is increasing pressure to "break the credentialing barrier" by emphasizing institutional accreditation instead of individual practitioner licensure. This trend is consistent with recent developments within the federal government. The Health Care Financing Administration (HCFA) has begun to remove specific mention of individual professional credentials in federal regulations pertaining to the Medicare program. The rationale is that hospitals and other health-care facilities should decide who is qualified to perform professional duties for their organizations.

The transdisciplinary team approach and the multicompetent health-practitioner movement present new opportunities as well as challenges for professional practice in the next 10 years. For either movement to be successful, current laws, regulations, and traditions must be carefully reviewed. Modifications should be made only after provisions have been made for public awareness of the possible limitations in knowledge and expertise of so-called multiskilled personnel. Nevertheless, there will probably continue to be room for both specialists and generalists in most fields. It will be important for all practitioners to develop more cost-efficient and effective models for service delivery to meet the changing needs of society, while at the same time maintaining professional integrity.

The Nonteam Practitioner

Is there life without a team? Obviously, not every speech-language pathologist will practice within the context of formal team approaches. Many of us never have access to a comprehensive service delivery environment; others have work arrangements in which they never really become part of a staff. For example, hospital speech-language pathology services in some areas are delivered under contract by a practitioner who travels to several facilities. There is little time for consultation with other professionals during treatment visits. The SLP may have to return to the hospital to attend team meetings or case staffings, for which he or she may not be paid. Under these circumstances, formal collaboration is very limited, but professional interaction is not impossible.

It takes initiative and creativity to devise ways of working cooperatively with other professionals when the organizational structure is not conducive to a team approach. Most other professionals probably will welcome an initial, exploratory contact with the speech-language pathologist. Perhaps a meeting can be convened to discuss ways of communicating regularly—if not in person, then by telephone, written report, or memorandum. Facility administrators may be very supportive of staff efforts to form a communication network, and a formal team structure could be an outgrowth of such early efforts. The speech-language pathologist can be a very appropriate initiator and facilitator of team building. The most important thing to remember is that quality patient care is the primary focus of our work. That task will be better served by overcoming obstacles to working successfully with the other professionals who serve our patients.

■ SUMMARY

In this chapter we have briefly described the credentials and roles of health and education professionals in today's human services sectors. Secondly, we discussed team approaches to patient care, highlighting current trends in service delivery. Finally, we suggested ways in which persons who do not participate in a formal team structure can facilitate interprofessional communication.

Opportunities for collaboration in human services are likely to expand as the demand to control the cost and utilization of services intensifies. Many of our readers will participate in a futher restructuring of the health and education systems that will present new challenges to all human service professionals to find more effective and efficient ways to serve individuals who need our help.

ACTIVITIES

1. Interview one of the professionals discussed in this chapter to learn more about her or his knowledge, skills, and interests; impressions about speech-language pathologists; and opinions about various treatment team approaches.

2. Observe treatment sessions conducted by other professionals. Ask a regular or special educator if you can observe a class.

3. Read articles in the professional journals published by the American Physical Therapy Association, American Medical Association, National Education Association, American Occupational Therapy Association, American Psychological Association, and the National Association of Social Workers. What seem to be the main concerns and issues addressed by these groups? How do they compare with ASHA's interests? How are the publications alike? How are they different?

4. Investigate the patient-care approaches used by hospitals and other health-care facilities in your area. It might be possible to interview a team coordinator, director of rehabilitation medicine, director of patient-care services, or director of communication disorders. In some cases you may be permitted to attend a team meeting.

5. Develop a model for patient care for your facility (university clinic, off-campus practicum site, etc.) based on one or more of the models discussed in this chapter. Consider the administrative structure of the facility or program, available resources, personnel, attitudes of staff members of various departments or clinics, practice patterns, and existing team efforts.

REFERENCES

American Occupational Therapy Association. (1979). *Uniform terminology for reporting occupational therapy services.* Rockville, MD: AOTA.

ASHA Committee on Language. (1987a). The role of speech-language pathologists in the habilitation and rehabilitation of cognitively-impaired individuals. *Asha, 29*(6), 53–55.

ASHA, Statement of the American Speech-Language-Hearing Association and the National Association of School Psychologists. (1987b). Position paper on language learning disorders. *Asha, 29*(3), 55–56.

ASHA Committee on Language, Speech and Hearing Services in Schools. (1984). Guidelines for caseload size for speech-language services in the schools. *Asha, 26*(4), 53–57.

Bamberg, R., & Blayney, K. (1984). Multicompetent allied health professionals: Current approaches and suggestions for baccalaureate level programs. *Allied Health, 13,* 229–305.

Blayney, K. (1986). Restructuring the health care labor force: The rise of the multiskilled allied health practitioner. *Alabama Journal of Medical Science, 23*(3), 277–278.

Clark, D. (1979). Health systems clerkship: Study guide and resource manual. University of Kentucky: University Press of Kentucky.

England, B. (Ed.). (1986). *Medical rehabilitation services in health care institutions.* Chicago: American Hospital Publishers.

Frassinelli, L., Superior, K., & Meyers, J. (1983). A consultation model for speech and language intervention. *Asha, 25*(1), 25–30.

Komaroff, A. (1985). Quality assurance in 1984. *Medical Care, 23*(5), 723–734.

Larkins, P., ASHA Professional Practice Division. (1986, Winter). *Update: Speech-Language Pathology Liaison Branch.* Rockville, MD: ASHA.

Lowe, J., & Herranen, M. (1978). Conflict in teamwork: Understanding roles and relationships. *Social Work in Health Care, 3*(3), 323–330.

Lugenbeel, A. (1986). Multiple competency: Its time is here. *Alabama Journal of Medical Science, 23*(3), 279–280.

McCormick, L., & Lee, C. (1979). Public Law 94–142: Mandated partnerships. *American Journal of Occupational Therapy, 33*(9), 586–588.

Melvin, J. (1980). Interdisciplinary and multidisciplinary activities and the American Congress of Rehabilitation Medicine. *Archives of Physical Medicine and Rehabilitation, 61,* 379–380.

Morgan, F. (1986). The nature of existing multicompetency programs. *Alabama Journal of Medical Science, 23*(3), 281–282.

Nelson, N. (1984). Beyond information processing: The language of teachers and textbooks. In G. Wallach and K. Butler (Eds.), *Language learning disabilities in school-age children* (pp. 154–178). Baltimore, MD: Williams & Wilkins.

————. (1985). Teacher talk and child listening: Fostering a better match. In C. Simon (Ed.), *Communication skills and classroom success: Assessment of language-learning disabled students* (pp. 65–104). San Diego, CA: College-Hill.

Pellegrino, E. (1977). The allied health professions: The problems and potentials of maturity. *Journal of Allied Health, 6,* 25–29.

Pickering, M. (1981). Consulting with the classroom teacher to promote language acquisition and usage. *Topics in Learning and Learning Disabilities, 1*(2), 59–68.

Simon, C. (Ed.). (1985). *Communication skills and classroom success: Therapy methodologies for language-learning disabled students.* San Diego, CA: College-Hill.

Stapp, J., Tucker, A., & VandenBos, G. (1985). Census of psychological personnel: 1983. *American Psychologist, 40*(12), 1317–1351.

Tomes, L. & Sanger, D. (1986). Attitudes of interdisciplinary team members toward speech-language services in public schools. *Language, Speech and Hearing Services in Schools, 17*(3), 230–240.

U.S. Office of the Federal Register. (1985, July 1). *Code of Federal Regulations* (34 CFR 300.1). Washington, DC: U.S. Government Printing Office.

Watkins, R. (1983). Medical rehabilitation in the present and a promise for the future. *Annals of the Academy of Medicine, 12*(3), 438–442.

————. (1984, February). Personal correspondence. Chicago, IL.

CHAPTER SEVEN

Introduction to Health-Care Financing

INTRODUCTION

Health-care financing is currently one of the nation's most compelling issues. According to the Health Care Financing Administration, a total of $458 billion was spent on health care in the United States in 1986. That figure equates to per capita costs of $1,837 for the year. Of the total amount spent on health care in 1986, federal, state, and local governments paid $189.7 billion, private insurance financed $140.7 billion, and consumers paid $116.1 billion through direct payments and insurance premiums. Personal health-care services constituted the largest proportion of expenditures, with hospital care and physician services leading all other categories by a wide margin. Overall, health expenditures increased 8.4% over 1985 totals.

During the 1970s, health-care costs escalated. Consequently, both the public and private sectors have initiated a wide variety of cost-containment strategies that include alternative financing and delivery mechanisms. Health care is no longer just a personal matter between the patient and a health professional of choice. Payors are no longer writing checks without question. Health care is becoming a complex, competitive business. Social policy questions are raised by the new focus on cost reductions. Health care as we know it today may be very different in the next 10 years; and even with cost restraints in place, health-care expenditures are expected to top $1.5 trillion by 2000.

Changes in the way health care is financed and delivered will have important implications for the clinical practice of speech-language pathology. This chapter is intended to be a readable, comprehensive, and understandable guide to private- and public-sector health-care financing and service delivery mechanisms, with emphasis on issues of special interest to speech-language pathologists.

GOVERNMENT HEALTH PROGRAMS

Medicare

Medicare is a federally sponsored health-insurance program for persons aged 65 and over and certain individuals under age 65 who are disabled or who have end-stage renal disease. Authorized under Title XVIII of the Social Security Act of 1965, Medicare is administered by the Health Care Financing Administration (HCFA) of the U.S. Department of Health and Human Services. HCFA contracts with fiscal intermediaries and carriers—Blue Cross/Blue Shield plans and commercial insurers predominantly—who perform day-to-day administrative functions such as determining reasonable costs and benefits for covered services, analyzing and processing claims, and making payments to providers.

Benefits are provided in two parts:

- Part A: Hospital insurance—covers inpatient services while beneficiaries are in hospitals, skilled-nursing facilities, or hospices, or receiving home health benefits.
- Part B: Supplementary medical insurance—covers physicians' services (inpatient or outpatient), laboratory services, outpatient rehabilitation services, medical equipment and supplies, treatment for end-stage renal disease, and certain other outpatient categories.

Part A is a mandatory program funded by a portion of the Social Security payroll tax (Federal Insurance Contribution Act—FICA). Beneficiaries also pay deductibles and copayments. Part B is a voluntary program for which beneficiaries pay a monthly premium. After payment of an annual deductible, Part B covers 80% of the cost of covered benefits. Part B premiums actually cover only about 24% of the costs of the program; the rest is subsidized through FICA taxes and the general fund. Over 95% of the nation's 31 million Medicare beneficiaries carry Part B coverage.

Total program costs for medicare in 1987 are expected to exceed $78 billion. Yet, there are still large gaps in coverage for which a beneficiary may incur substantial financial losses. For example, in 1987 a deductible of $520 is required for each "spell of illness" under Part A. Copayments are also required if a hospital stay exceeds 60 days, and no benefits are paid after a 90-day stay, if the lifetime reserve of 60 days is exhausted. Skilled-nursing-facility (SNF) benefits are provided only if the patient has spent at least three days in an acute-care hospital and is transferred to the SNF. Medicare pays the full cost of the first 20 days; the beneficiary pays a copayment for days 21 through 100, after which no benefits are paid.

According to the Congressional Budget Office, 72% of Medicare beneficiaries buy so-called Medigap insurance from private insurance companies to protect themselves from potential losses. About half of these policies are purchased individually and half by the retirees' former employers under group-benefits plans. These plans are highly variable in quality but typically cover some or all of the deductibles and copayments, and may cover certain other services not covered by Medicare. The Baucus Amendments to the Social Security Act (PL 96–265) established minimum standards for state regulation and voluntary certification of Medigap policies. Still, there is considerable controversy about the way these policies are marketed and the extent to which they cover potential losses. The responsibility of the private sector and federal government in meeting the high costs of catastrophic illnesses is currently being debated by Congress. Some resolution of the issue will probably occur through reform of the Medicare program in the near future.

A major Medicare reform took place in 1983 with the inception of the Prospective Payment System (PPS). Prior to that year, Medicare paid hospitals according to a cost-based method. Facilities were reimbursed for the reasonable costs they incurred in providing services to Medicare beneficiaries. Under that system, Medicare expenditures for hospital care, the largest and most expensive component of the program, soared. In response to the inability of the program to contain costs, the PPS was developed. Now, hospitals are prospectively paid set amounts of money, based upon patient classifications by diagnosis related groups (DRGs).

Each DRG grouping includes a set of diagnoses that require about the same amount of hospital resources for patient treatment. If a hospital can treat a patient for less money than Medicare pays for that patient's illness classification, the hospital is permitted to retain the remainder. The hospital must absorb any costs that exceed the amount Medicare pays. Patients can be charged only the usual deductible and copayments. All services, including speech-language pathology and audiology, rendered to acute-care inpatients are included in the prospective rate under Part A benefits.

The following inpatient settings are exempt from the PPS and continue to bill under the cost-based system: rehabilitation hospitals and distinct rehabilitation units within acute-care hospitals, long-term-care facilities, Veterans Administration hospitals, and children's hospitals. Part B services are billed according to so-called usual, customary, and reasonable (UCR) charges and are also exempt from PPS. Consequently, the emphasis in health care is shifting to alternative- and outpatient-care settings for which services may be billed separately. Rehabilitation services are being rendered increasingly in non-acute-care settings such as skilled-nursing facilities, rehabilitation hospitals and units, and through home health-care programs.

Speech-language pathology services have been part of the Medicare program since its inception. SLP services are rendered by qualified providers (licensed and certified or CFY) to eligible beneficiaries in Medicare-certified-provider settings: hospitals, skilled-nursing facilities, physician's offices, public health agencies, hospital outpatient clinics, home health agencies, comprehensive outpatient rehabilitation facilities, rehabilitation agencies, hospices, and recently, health maintenance organizations.

According to Medicare's speech-language pathology guidelines, SLP services are those services necessary for the diagnosis and treatment of speech and language disorders that result in communication disabilities. The services must relate directly to a written plan of treatment established by a physician or speech-language pathologist who works with the patient, and the need for services must be recertified by a physician every 30 days (60 days for a comprehensive outpatient rehabilitation facility). Additionally, services must be "reasonable and necessary," in accordance with the following stipulations:

1. The services must be considered under accepted standards of practice to be a specific and effective treatment for the patient's condition.
2. The services must be of such a level of complexity and sophistication or the patient's condition must be such that the services required can be effectively performed only by or under the supervision of a qualified speech-language pathologist.
3. There must be an expectation that the patient's condition will improve significantly in a reasonable period of time.
4. The amount, frequency, and duration of the services must be reasonable under accepted standards of practice.

Speech-language pathologists who provide services to Medicare beneficiaries are either employees of a facility or program, or they deliver services by contractual arrangement with Medicare-certified-provider types. Currently, the two provider types for which an individual speech-language pathologist may obtain his or her own Medicare provider number are the rehabilitation agency (RA) or comprehensive outpatient rehabilitation facility (CORF). A RA can be established by either a SLP or physical therapist who also includes social or vocational adjustment services as needed in the rehabilitation program (usually under contract with a social worker or other counselor). The RA provides "an integrated multidisciplinary program designed to upgrade the physical functioning of the handicapped, disabled individual by bringing together as a team specialized rehabilitation personnel" (42 CFR 405.1702). A CORF is a nonresidential facility established for the purpose of providing diagnostic, therapeutic, and restorative services to ill, injured, or disabled outpatients. The plan of treatment must be established by a physician for all services (unlike other provider types). Core services required for certification as a CORF include physician's services, physical therapy, and social or psychological services. Speech-language pathology services are among additional services that may be included in a CORF program.

White (1986a) offers succinct assistance for SLPs who are considering establishing a CORF or RA. He states that the primary decision between the two provider types hinges on whether the practitioner can provide services in a multitude of settings or have the ability to be reimbursed for a multitude of services at one site. RA practitioners may provide services in an office, nursing home, or the patient's home, but reimbursement is restricted to speech-language pathology services, physical therapy, and administrative costs. Social work or vocational services are not directly reimbursable. Conversely, all CORF services are reimbursed but must be delivered at the facility.

Speech-language pathologists who have Medicare provider numbers will communicate primarily with a Medicare carrier who will accept, process, and pay claims. Medicare regional offices issue manuals and transmittals (see the glossary at the end of this chapter) to apprise intermediaries, carriers, and providers of Medicare policies and procedures. Regional offices may be contacted if a practitioner is experiencing problems with an intermediary or carrier. The central office of the Health Care Financing Administration is in Baltimore, Maryland.

Medicare is an ever-evolving, controversial, and political program. Each administration and Congress has its own agenda for Medicare reform. The current issues include expansion of the Medicare program to help beneficiaries cover catastrophic-illness expenses and the privatization of the program. Medicare's Private Health Plan Option (PHPO) is discussed in the "Health Maintenance Organization" section of this chapter.

Medicaid

Authorized by Title XIX of the Social Security Act, the Medicaid program provides grants to states to fund health-care services for low-income persons. Eligibility for the program is generally based on whether one qualifies to receive payments under public assistance programs such as Aid to Families with Dependent Children (AFDC) or Supplemental Security Income (SSI), but there are also other categories under which a person may establish eligibility. About 13% of Medicare beneficiaries also qualify to receive Medicaid benefits. This situation is referred to as *dual entitlement*. State Medicaid programs may pay the recipient's Medicare premium for Part B as well as the deductibles and coinsurance for both Parts A and B.

The original intent of the Medicaid program at its inception in 1965 was to pay for the medical care for low-income women and children. Indeed, of the approximately 23 million recipients, 10.3 million are children under 12, and 5.9 million are adults in AFDC families. The remainder include 3 million persons aged 65 and over, 3.2 million blind and disabled individuals, and 3 million persons in other categories. However, proportional expenditures do not match recipient status. Seventy-five percent of program expenditures go for care of the elderly and disabled. Institutional long-term care composes the largest portion of the Medicaid budget. It funds almost half of the nursing-home care in this country (see Figure 7.1). The other half of expenses are paid by patients or their families.

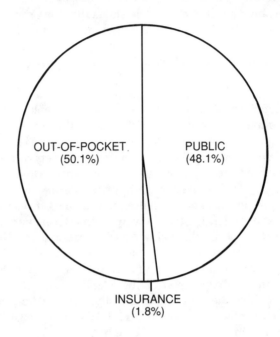

FIGURE 7.1
Sources of Payment for Long-Term Care
NOTE: From Health Care Financing Administration, Office of the Actuary, 1984.

In order to qualify for Medicaid, the nursing-home resident must "spend down," which means that the person must become impoverished according to Medicaid eligibility levels. If there is a noninstitutionalized spouse, that person must then live in poverty. With annual nursing-home costs averaging $25,000, it does not take long for most persons to deplete their life savings. Private long-term-care insurance is available, but only a small segment of the population has coverage. As the need for coverage becomes more publicized, the market for such insurance is expected to grow rapidly.

Within broad federal guidelines, states have considerable flexibility to determine the extent of Medicaid benefits offered as well as fee schedules. Only a few services are mandatory:

1. Inpatient and outpatient hospital care;
2. Physicians' services;
3. Health screening services for children under 21;
4. Skilled-nursing-facility services and certain home health services for persons over 21.

States may also cover a broad range of additional services including care in intermediate-care facilities (ICF), pharmaceuticals, prosthetic devices, and rehabilitation services in settings other than hospitals and skilled-nursing facilities (SNF). Speech-language pathology services are included in the services required for reimbursement in hospitals and SNFs but are optional services in other settings. Because the programs vary from state to state, practitioners should contact the state Medicaid agency to receive specific information about coverage and reimbursement.

Medicaid is following the rest of the health-care system in its move toward cost containment and managed care. In 1986 federal contributions to Medicare exceeded $25 million; state and local governments contributed an additional $18 million to fund their portion of the Medicaid program. The federal government is expected to limit its contribution to Medicaid, thereby encouraging states to adopt new methods of cost management. Through freedom-of-choice or home- and community-based waiver systems, states are developing alternative health-care-delivery mechanisms such as case-management and utilization-review requirements or enrollment of Medicaid recipients in health maintenance organizations (HMOs).

The Medicaid program is becoming increasingly complex and controversial as the nation attempts to address the issues of long-term care and access to quality health care for all citizens. Friedman (1987) provides an excellent summary of Medicaid's problems:

> It is supposed to cover the care of welfare mothers and children, blind people, disabled individuals and the low-income elderly—a highly heterogeneous constituency. It is constantly torn between acute care and the requirements of the chronically ill. It is financed by the federal government, states, and some counties, leading to a labyrinth of eligibility, coverage, and payment policies. Some states have generous eligibility standards; others bare bones. Some cover little more than required services whereas others offer a wide range. With varied and, to a large extent, mutually exclusive constituencies that often share only their political powerlessness, Medicaid is far too fragmented to have a strong political identity. (p. 51)

Congress is currently debating long-term-care funding issues. Over the next decade, funding for long-term care may be shifted to the Medicare program and private insurance. The budget for Medicaid may then be used for its original intent.

Other Government Programs

Civilian Health and Medical Program of the Uniformed Services (CHAMPUS)

CHAMPUS is a medical benefits program provided by the federal government through the Department of Defense to pay for health care rendered to the following persons: spouses and dependents of uniformed services personnel; retired uniformed services personnel and their spouses and dependents; and the spouses and dependents of deceased uniformed services personnel. The uniformed services include the U.S. Army, Navy, Air Force, Marine Corp, Coast Guard, Commissioned Corp of the United States Public Health Service, and Commissioned Corp of the National Oceanic and Atmospheric Administration.

The Office of CHAMPUS (OCHAMPUS), located in Denver, Colorado, contracts with private organizations to process and pay claims. There are approximately 6 million CHAMPUS beneficiaries who pay deductibles and copayments, but no premiums. Although beneficiaries are encouraged to obtain all necessary care at uniformed services medical facilities, they may seek care from civilian sources in certain cases. Institutional and individual health providers must be authorized by CHAMPUS to render services to CHAMPUS beneficiaries.

CHAMPUS is currently in a transitional period as it begins a phase-in period of privatizing the program. On an experimental basis CHAMPUS is awarding contracts to private health-care organizations and professionals to provide health care to beneficiaries for a set fee paid by CHAMPUS.

Speech-language pathology and audiology services are covered when prescribed by a physician and rendered as part of a treatment addressed to a physical defect, but not to any educational or occupational deficit. Coverage includes treatment for communication disorders related to cerebral palsy, congenital defects, stroke, brain injury, vocal cord surgery, repeated ear infections that interfere with speech development, and significant hearing loss (Downey, White, & Karr, 1984).

Veterans Administration

The Veterans Administration (VA) provides an integrated system of health services for a potential pool of 28 million military veterans of the uniformed services. The core of the system is a network of 172 Veterans Administration Medical Centers (VAMC) across the United States, although the VA also contracts with other individual providers and institutions to provide care for eligible veterans. The VAMCs have a total bed capacity of 80,000. VA medical services include inpatient and outpatient care, institutional and noninstitutional long-term care, and other specialized programs. All VA medical centers provide comprehensive speech-language pathology and audiology services. Professionals who work in these centers also participate in the VA's extensive health professional's training programs as well as medical research projects. In 1986, Congress revised the eligibility requirements for participation in VA medical programs under Public Law 99–272. There are now three eligibility categories based upon both financial and nonfinancial criteria. Only Category C veterans are required to make copayments for care rendered.

PRIVATE-SECTOR HEALTH-CARE FINANCING AND SERVICE DELIVERY

The private health insurance industry is integral to the financing of health care in the United States. A larger share of benefits is paid by private insurers than the combined spending of the Medicare and Medicaid programs and direct payments by patients. Most private insurance is obtained as an employee benefit and is a major employer expense (Farley, 1986). Arnett and Trapnell (1984) define private health insurance as "insurance that pays for the costs of preventing, diagnosing, or treating an accident, illness, pregnancy, or other health condition requiring medical related services" (p. 36). There are other types of insurance that are related to health care, including short- and long-term disability, accidental death and dismemberment, and automobile-accident coverage, but our discussion is limited to benefits payable upon the provision of a specific medical or related service.

Private health insurance can be classified into several categories: commercial insurance, Blue Cross/Blue Shield, and independent plans (e.g., self-insured employers, union plans, HMOs). The distinctions among the categories are not easily defined as the insurance industry diversifies and integrates services. Insurance companies have become major sponsors or cosponsors of HMOs and PPOs. They offer administrative services and stop-loss or reinsurance coverage for self-insured employers and utilization review services for all clients. Large hospital chains are buying insurance companies, and they may offer an HMO and PPO as well as traditional coverage. The health insurance industry is clearly complex, but in the following discussion we attempt to provide a comprehensive overview of the health insurance and new service delivery mechanisms as they exist in a rapidly changing environment.

Commercial Health Insurance

Health insurance is based on the concept of risk. Insurance companies base their premiums—the amount paid by policyholders for coverage—on actuarial data. An actuary is a professional who calculates the risk of incurring illnesses or injuries according to individual and aggregate variables related to age, sex, occupation, and other demographic data in addition to prevalence and incidence rates for various diseases, medical conditions, and accidents. The company bases its decision to insure someone and how much to charge for coverage on the likelihood that the person will get sick or sustain an injury. Premiums are usually experience rated, which means that the amount charged is based on the average cost of actual or anticipated care used by various groups of subscribers. Because some subscribers will submit many claims and others will submit very few, insurance companies are able to spread the risk across all policyholders. The reason group health insurance plan premiums are less costly than individual coverage is that the risk to the insurance company is spread over a larger population with group plans.

An insurance policy is a contract in which the insurer agrees to pay the policyholder for losses related to designated contingencies. In order to protect the insurance company against the costs associated with a large volume of claims, the insurer stipulates the conditions for coverage. The company usually will not cover preexisting conditions (that is, health problems the insured already had when the policy was purchased) and there is often a waiting period for eligibility for certain benefits. In addition, there are often annual and/or lifetime dollar limitations on the amount the company will pay for a person's health problem. Policies also exclude or restrict certain conditions and/or providers of services.

Insurance companies usually cover benefits for which subscribers (usually employers) are willing to pay the premiums and for which it is possible to determine the risk of needing the benefit. They typically offer different types and levels of benefits according to the agreement negotiated between the insurer and the purchaser. Contracts are highly variable. A large company may offer hundreds of different plans, including HMO and PPO options. In addition to basic, major medical, and comprehensive major medical plans, there are single-benefit riders and special policies for things like dental care. Recently, insurance companies have begun to offer policies that insure against the high costs associated with institutional and noninstitutional long-term care.

There are more than 800 commercial insurance companies covering 100 million persons. Insurers are regulated by state insurance codes in all states and the District of Columbia. These regulations establish standards for financial solvency, surpluses and reserves (see the glossary) and investments; license insurance brokers and agents; and regulate claims processing, grievance procedures, advertising, premium rating, and policy content. Many states also have mandated that certain benefits be included in all insurance policies written in that state. Mandates can be divided into three basic categories for coverage of (1) specific services, (2) particular groups of dependents such as newborns or divorced spouses, and (3) certain health-care provider groups, for example nurse practitioners or psychologists (Demkovich, 1986). The services of speech-language pathologists and audiologists are mandated optional benefits in Arkansas, Missouri, and Texas; legislation is pending in other states.

The employer community, primarily through the business coalition movement (see the glossary) has put pressure on the insurance industry to hold down rising premium costs and help control utilization of services. Employers are increasingly asking employees to pay higher deductibles and copayments and are directing employees to specific providers and plans through PPO and HMO structures. Consequently, insurance companies have become major sponsors or cosponsors of HMOs and PPOs. They offer administrative services only (ASO) and stop-loss or reinsurance (see the glossary) coverage for self-insured employers as well as utilization review services for all clients. As part of the cost-containment movement, insurers, consulting firms, and managed-care companies are selling "managed-care" services. Managed care is a system for determining medical necessity and cost effectiveness of services provided by health professionals and facilities. The core of managed care is utilization review, a system used to evaluate the necessity, appropriateness, and efficiency of health-care services. Reviews are conducted before service (prospectively), during service (concurrently), and after service (retrospectively). Some components of utilization review (UR) include preadmission certification or preauthorization, second opinion, claim and bill auditing, discharge planning, and medical case management. Case management is a system for coordinating services for high-cost cases (e.g., stroke, spinal cord and head injuries) that require intensive and/or long-term services. Case-management services are offered by insurance companies, consulting firms, managed-care companies, and provider groups. Case management presents some interesting challenges for the health-care community, and it may be a very positive step for rehabilitation services. There is a growing trend for insurers to include rehabilitation services in case-management programs that are not specifically covered in regular plans. More information about managed care can be found in Cornett (1987).

As health care moves from an emphasis upon acute inpatient care to outpatient and alternative-care programs, insurers are changing the type and level of benefits offered to meet changing needs. The intent is to reduce patients' needs for intensive and prolonged care by encouraging preventive, maintenance, and restorative care. Insurers and other plans do this by paying for routine and prophylactic care, rehabilitation services, and the services of less costly but effective and efficient nonphysician health-care providers. The insurance industry is a long way from fulfilling this goal, but the structure of coverage is beginning to change.

Coverage of speech-language pathology services by commercial insurers depends on the provisions written in an individual's insurance contract. Most clients are covered under group health benefits plans negotiated between an employer and the insurer. If included, speech-language pathology services are usually incorporated in major medical or supplementary plans or riders rather than basic benefits. It is likely that restrictions and exclusions apply. Services are typically covered for communication disorders caused by illness or accidents but not developmental problems. Congenital disorders, such as treatment for communication problems associated with cleft palate, may be covered. Some companies require physician prescription or referral for speech-language pathology services. Other companies only require that a licensed professional provide the service. In states that do not license speech-language pathologists and audiologists, ASHA certification is often accepted. White (1986b) has addressed the issue of licensure and third-party reimbursement elsewhere.

Coverage for audiology services is less variable than for speech-language pathology. Nearly all companies cover audiologic testing ordered by a physician to establish a medical diagnosis. Other types of evaluations may not be covered, however, and hearing aids are usually specifically excluded.

The Health Insurance Association of America (HIAA) issued a report in 1986 to its member insurance companies that outlined the professional qualifications, continuing education practices, and professional services rendered by speech-language pathologists and audiologists. The report specifically stated that "there is no requirement for medical prescription or supervision since the profession is autonomous." (State licensure laws also address the issue.) Copies of the HIAA report are available from the ASHA National Office. More detailed information about speech-language pathology and audiology and insurance companies is found in Downey, White, and Karr (1984), and Chwat and Gurland (1984).

Blue Cross/Blue Shield

In 1929 the prototype for health-service benefits in the United States was established when Baylor University negotiated an agreement with a hospital in Dallas, Texas, to provide care for a group of teachers for a prepaid fee. This type of arrangement was gradually adopted by organizations in other locations across the country and came to be known as Blue Cross. Blue Shield was an outgrowth of the medical prepayment bureaus that existed in the late 1800s. The first Blue Shield plan was formed in California in 1939. Today, there are 78 independent Blue Cross/Blue Shield plans, with an enrollment of more than 76 million persons. Blue Cross covers hospital benefits, and Blue Shield pays for the services of physicians and other health-care professionals. Most BC/BS plans have become joint corporations.

The plans are voluntary, nonprofit health-service corporations that contract directly with health-care providers to deliver services on a prepaid basis to subscribers. Thus, BC/BS primarily offers service benefits—not dollars—to patients. Participating providers bill BC/BS directly and are usually paid according to a usual, customary, and reasonable (UCR) mechanism, and the providers accept BC/BS payment as payment in full. The patient, however, pays applicable deductibles and copayments. Nonparticipating providers are paid according to a fee schedule for certain medical-surgical procedures. In these cases, the patient must pay the provider the difference between charges and the set fee, unless the patient's annual income falls below a certain level. Patients may obtain care from nonparticipating providers but may have to make full payment to the provider initially and be reimbursed later by the BC/BS plan. Nonparticipating providers may, of course, charge patients more than what BC/BS pays for the services.

Although independent, BC/BS plans are organized as a nationwide federation of autonomous plans, and they are usually subject to state insurance regulations. Until recently, plans were exempt from federal income taxes. Many BC/BS plans do have for-profit subsidiaries and affiliates; a number of plans also sell life insurance. In addition, BC/BS plans have become one of the largest sponsors of HMOs and PPOs in the country. Through the Blue Cross/Blue Shield Association, the BC/BS coordinating agency headquartered in Chicago, BC/BS is the primary intermediary/carrier for the Medicare program. Like commercial insurers, BC/BS plans tailor benefit packages to meet the specific needs of subscribers. Thus, there is no typical coverage or premium rate. Benefits and benefit levels are commensurate with what the subscriber is willing to purchase. More than 90% of BC/BS business is employer-sponsored group coverage.

Most Blue Shield plans cover the services of certain nonphysician health-care providers, such as dentists, optometrists, podiatrists, chiropractors, psychologists, and physical therapists. Speech-language pathologists and audiologists are sometimes among those professionals approved for either direct or indirect reimbursement. Certain plans require that SLP services be supervised by a physician, whereas others stipulate that physicians must refer patients to speech-language pathologists. Other plans have no requirements for supervision or referral. Like commercial insurers, BC/BS generally provides benefits for communication disorders that are related to medical conditions. Two plans that illustrate current trends in coverage of SLP services in Blue Cross/Blue Shield policies are BC/BS of Maine and BC/BS of Maryland.

Maine's SLP benefit was established in its major-medical plan in 1983. Physicians must refer patients to a licensed speech-language pathologist. SLP is defined as treatment for correction of a communication impairment resulting from illness, disease, trauma, or congenital anomaly that results in the restoration or improvement of lost functions. SLP services are limited to 30 sessions per patient per calendar year, unless further services are medically necessary. Professionals are reimbursed according to the usual, customary, and reasonable (UCR) method. BC/BS of Maryland added a speech-language pathology benefit to their Gold Standard Plan in 1986. Coverage is provided for outpatient SLP services for rehabilitation of a speech/language disorder resulting from disease, trauma, or physical disorder. According to the benefit, language rehabilitation is "the coordinated use of medical and therapeutic means in order to restore a physical or intellectual function impaired by disease or trauma; maintain progress achieved during treatment, and prevent regression." The function must "significantly improve" in an observable way within a reasonable time period. Coverage for SLP services extends to 50 outpatient visits per year. After the first 10 visits a treatment plan must be authorized by the BC/BS Outpatient Pretreatment Certification Program. Reauthorization is required in 10-visit increments up to 50 visits. Independent practitioners may be reimbursed directly and must have individual BC/BS provider numbers. It is likely that more BC/BS plans will add speech-language pathology and audiology benefits with precertification and utilization review program controls as part of a national managed-care trend for all health services.

Health Maintenance Organizations

Health maintenance organization (HMO) is a term first used in 1970 to describe a prepaid system of health care that focuses on using resources to maintain health rather than just to treat illnesses. Prepaid medical-service plans in the United States have existed since the 1800s, but the contemporary HMO originated in the late 1920s in response to lack of available medical services for groups of workers in the western states.

In 1973, Congress passed the HMO Act (PL 93–222), which defined health maintenance organizations and specified qualifications and regulations for HMO organization and development. A HMO is a legal entity that provides directly or arranges for basic and supplemental health-care services for a voluntarily enrolled population in a certain geographic area. HMOs are different from the third-party reimbursement system in that they combine the financing and delivery of health care in one organization. In addition, one fee, called a capitation, paid on a monthly or annual basis, covers all necessary services.

HMOs may be publicly or privately owned and are sponsored by insurance companies, business firms, health-care providers, labor unions, consumer groups, and other organizations. For-profit plans comprise the majority of the almost 800 HMOs in operation, and approximately 30 million persons are now enrolled in HMOs. Just under 60% of HMOs are federally qualified, which means they must meet specific requirements stated in the HMO Act as well as the regulations issued by the Health Care Financing Administration's Office of Prepaid Health-Care.

HMOs are organized according to four models: staff, group, independent practice association (IPA), and network. Figure 7.2 contains a summary of these structures. The most popular model is the IPA, followed by network, group, and staff models. The IPA is especially appealing to both enrollees and health professionals because it retains some of the characteristics of the traditional practitioner-patient relationship, including a modified fee-for-service payment system and patient visits to an individual provider's office.

To control utilization and channel enrollees to appropriate services, HMOs use a gatekeeper system. The gatekeeper is a health professional, usually a primary-care physician or nurse practitioner, who must authorize all elective admissions to a hospital, referrals to specialists, use of ancillary services, and certain other tests and procedures. Because one fee is supposed to cover all or most of enrollees' health-care needs, there is a built-in incentive for the HMO to keep patients out of hospitals. Thus, HMO enrollees under age 65 spend far fewer days in the hospitals than other patients. Inpatient days per 1,000 HMO enrollees for 1986 were 456. The national average was 957 days per 1,000 persons. When

FIGURE 7.2
Model Types

Staff
Health-care providers are salaried employees of the HMO and practice at a central facility.

Group
A multispecialty physician group practice contracts with a HMO to provide health services in their own offices or sometimes at a central facility.

Individual Practice Association (IPA)
HMO contracts with individual health-care practitioners to provide services to enrollees in their own offices. Providers may be paid on a fee-for-service or capitated basis.

Network
HMO contracts with both multispeciality groups and individual health professionals to provide services to enrollees. Networks usually involve a larger number of providers and may cover multiple geographic areas.

HMO enrollees were hospitalized, their average length of stay (LOS) was 4.5 days, compared to a national average of 5.5 days. The overall HMO concept is to keep people healthy by encouraging prevention and health maintenance. Unlike most other health insurance plans, HMOs cover ongoing outpatient care, including well-baby visits, immunizations, and adult physical exams in basic benefits. Enrollees pay few or no out-of-pocket costs for these services.

Opponents of the HMO concept contend that HMOs may undertreat enrollees; proponents maintain that the system increases continuity, efficiency, and effectiveness of care. Quality of care, however, is not determined by volume or intensity of services, and there is evidence that traditional fee-for-service medicine may actually reward overservicing. To date, very few studies have concluded that HMOs provide poorer quality care than other health systems, but the debate will continue for years to come.

The status of speech-language pathology services in HMOs is somewhat difficult to determine. We are just beginning to collect data on the availability and utilization of rehabilitation services in these organizations. According to the HMO Act, federally qualified HMOs must provide or arrange for

> outpatient services and inpatient hospital services [which] shall include short-term rehabilitation and physical therapy, the provision of which the HMO determines can be expected to result in the significant improvement of a member's condition within a period of two months. (Code of Federal Regulations, 42 CFR, 110.102)

Cornett and Chabon (1986) conducted a survey of 47 HMOs across the country. Results suggested that most respondents limit speech-language pathology services to 60 days or two months. Consistent with traditional health insurance plans, communication disorders covered were generally problems related to illnesses or accidents. On the other hand, over 50% of the HMOs said they cover speech-language pathology services for disorders thought to be of a developmental, behavioral, or psychosocial etiology. Respondents indicated that SLP services are predominantly provided to HMOs by contractual agreement (54%) or informal arrangement (34%), with 12% employing salaried speech-language pathologists.

The Group Health Association of America (GHAA), a major trade association for HMOs, conducted a survey of their members in 1986 to obtain data related to 1985. The GHAA survey included 203 plans, representing a total enrollment of 14 million persons. All types of organizational models and geographic regions were represented, and both federally qualified and nonqualified HMOs participated. Only 8.9% of the respondents did not cover any speech-language pathology services, 28.6% placed no time restrictions or copayments on SLP services, and 13.3% had both limits and copayments. Limits only were required by 41.4% of the respondents, and copayments only by 7.9%. It is important to note that HMOs enrolling Medicare beneficiaries must provide or arrange for services in accordance with the Medicare statute. Thus, the limitations and copayments imposed on SLP services for other enrollees do not apply to Medicare HMO enrollees.

Since January 1985, when final regulations of the Tax Equity and Fiscal Responsibility Act of 1982 (TEFRA) were published, about 1.87 million Medicare beneficiaries have enrolled in federally qualified HMOs or competitive medical plans (see the glossary) that have risk contracts with the Health Care Financing Administration. A risk contract means that the HMO or competitive medical plan (CMP) has agreed to provide all necessary services to which Medicare beneficiaries are entitled in return for a flat fee paid by HCFA. The capitation plan, or Private Health Plan Option (PHPO), for Medicare beneficiaries is expected to expand to include employer- and union-sponsored retiree benefit programs as well as private insurance plans. Under an employer-based health-care plan (EBP), Medicare benefits would be combined with company-paid copayments in one integrated system. The companies or unions would receive fixed payments from the government in return for providing complete health coverage for Medicare-eligible retirees. HCFA is currently conducting demonstration projects to determine the feasibility of such arrangements. HCFA has also been conducting four demonstration programs in Oregon, New York, Minnesota, and California to test the feasibility of the Social HMO (SHMO) concept. The SHMO assumes responsibility for providing a full range of acute, rehabilitation, long-term, and personal-care services to voluntarily enrolled elderly persons for a prepaid fee, financed by a pooling of public- and private-sector resources. The SHMO is offered as one solution to the problem of paying for long-term care in this country.

HMOs are expected to continue to grow rapidly in the next decade, perhaps to a total enrollment of over 50 million. But the HMO concept may evolve into something quite different from today's HMO. Consolidations, mergers, and vertical integration will likely be the key to future HMO development, coupled with a trend toward offering multiple insurance products under one umbrella organization. A summary of HMO trends for the 1990s is presented in Figure 7.3.

Within this changing environment speech-language pathology and other rehabilitation services are likely to experience increased demand in HMOs. However, these services will be scrutinized to determine the overall cost/benefit ratio. SLPs who can offer an innovative range of services within more than one geographic area will be in a very good position to contract with HMOs. Also, there seems to be a growing trend toward formation of nonphysician Independent Practice Associations in which groups of individual practitioners such as dentists, speech-language pathologists, audiologists, physical therapists, and others contract with a HMO to provide services to their enrollees. In this way the IPA can institute peer-review systems to assist the HMO in controlling and monitoring utilization of services.

As the alternative delivery system evolves, differences between its two major components, HMOs and PPOs, are becoming increasingly blurred as the two plans respond to heightened competition. Preferred provider organizations may become even more successful than HMOs in the next decade.

Preferred Provider Organizations

Preferred provider organizations (PPOs) are contractual arrangements in which a selected group of health-care providers agree to deliver services to a specified

FIGURE 7.3
HMO Trends for the 1990s

- Hybrid plans
  HMOs will offer PPOs and indemnity options.
- Consolidations and mergers
  HMOs will emphasize national and regional plans and partnerships; commercial insurance–HMO joint ventures will arise.
- Vertical integration
  HMOs will acquire home health agencies, long-term-care facilities, surgicenters, emergicenters, ambulatory care clinics, durable medical equipment vendors, hospitals, and physical therapy and other rehabilitation practices.
- Diversity of products and benefit levels
  HMOs will offer dental and vision care,
  drug and alcohol rehabilitation,
  medical rehabilitation services,
  home-care and long-term-care options, and
  worker's compensation packages.
- Enrollment of special populations
  HMOs will enroll Medicare beneficiaries and
  Medicaid recipients.
- Emphasis on internal and external quality review

group of patients. Providers are paid predominantly on a fee-for-service basis according to a fee schedule or a discounting method. Although patients are usually not required to visit the "preferred" providers (except when enrolled in an exclusive provider organization—EPO), reduced-cost-sharing or enhanced-benefits incentives encourage patients to utilize the select panel. According to the American Medical Care and Review Association, 38 million persons have the option of obtaining health care through a PPO. In mid 1987 there were 535 operational PPOs and another 35 under development. Some analysts predict that 40% of all Americans will participate in a PPO in 10 years. PPO "enrollment" is difficult to quantify because PPOs are usually options within a regular health-insurance plan or other health program.

PPOs can be operated on a for-profit or a not-for-profit basis and are sponsored by health-care providers, entrepreneurs, or payers. Table 7.1 contains information on the various options for PPO sponsorship. Provider-sponsored PPOs bring together providers who are willing to participate in PPO arrangements but cannot themselves have enrollees. This type of PPO is similar to an IPA-model HMO in that the providers market their services to payer- or broker-sponsored PPOs or self-insured employers. In broker-sponsored PPOs the broker receives administrative fees from the payer and/or providers for managing and monitoring

TABLE 7.1
PPO Sponsorship

Provider	Broker/Entrepreneur	Payor
hospitals	private investors	Blue Cross/Blue Shield plans
hospital-physicians joint venture	third-party administrator (TPA)	commercial insurers
physician groups	utilization-review organizations	self-insured employers
nonphysician health professionals		union trust funds

the PPO network. Broker services typically include contracting, utilization review, and claims administration. Payer-sponsored PPOs select a panel of preferred providers and monitor utilization and management of health-care resources. There is a growing trend toward joint provider-insurer sponsorship of PPOs.

The intent of the PPO arrangement is to channel patients to cost-efficient providers. The PPO is the liaison between the sponsor, patients, and subcontractors. Cost-control mechanisms center on strict utilization review procedures, including preadmission certification, second surgical opinions, concurrent and retrospective reviews, and practice-pattern profiles among the preferred providers. Thus far, PPOs have achieved 15% to 20% cost savings over traditional fee-for-service plans through selective contracting, utilization review requirements, and prospectively determined payment mechanisms and discounting. The complexities of PPO arrangements are depicted in Figure 7.4. Twenty-two states currently have enabling statutes or regulations that govern the activities of PPOs.

PPOs have always incorporated some of the characteristics of HMOs, but there have been distinct differences. For example, PPO enrollees retain freedom of choice, but at a higher cost. HMOs assume financial risk for high utilization of service, whereas PPOs place the risk on the purchasers. PPOs use the fee-for-service system to pay providers; HMOs favor capitation (fixed payments). Unlike HMOs, PPOs need not be a specific legal entity but can be a network of contractual arrangements.

These distinctions are beginning to blur, however, as the development of hybrid HMOs and PPOs occurs. New types of organizations are emerging in which PPO providers share financial risk; a "gatekeeper" is used as a utilization control in PPOs; and HMOs allow enrollees to seek services outside the plan, as PPOs now do. The picture is further complicated by development of triple-option group insurance plans whereby employees are offered the choice of a regular indemity plan, PPO, or HMO under a single administrative and pricing mechanism. These plans are consistent with the movement toward flexible employee-

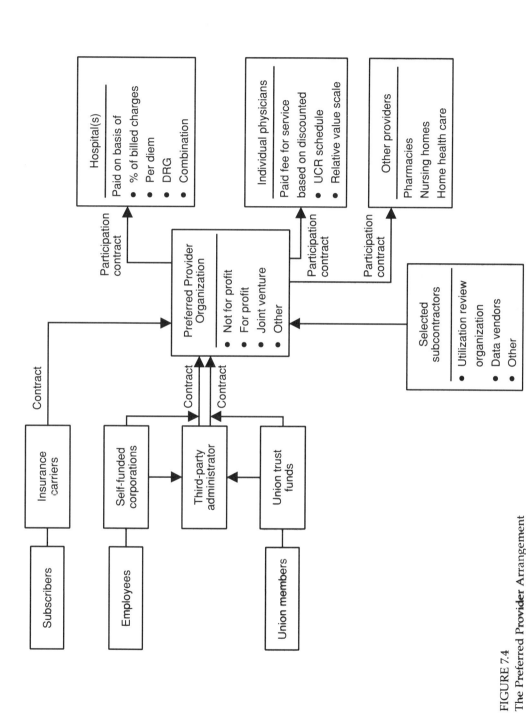

FIGURE 7.4
The Preferred Provider Arrangement

NOTE: From The PPO Handbook by S. Barger, D. Hillman, and H. Garland, 1985, Rockville, MD: Aspen Systems. Reprinted with permission of Aspen Publishers, Inc. Copyright 1985.

benefits plans. According to Fox and Anderson (1986), "the organization that is purely a HMO or PPO may be a relic of the past" (p. 27). In order for providers and insurers to protect and expand their market share in today's competitive environment, they are increasingly offering services through multiple organizational structures. An outline of PPO trends for the next decade appears in Figure 7.5.

It is difficult to determine the extent of speech-language pathologists' involvement in PPOs because no current data are available. As private practice among speech-language pathologists expands, these professionals will probably increase their contracting in these types of arrangements and organizations. Additionally, hospital departments and clinics may be part of hospital-sponsored PPOs. The PPO seems to be a viable practice option for nonphysician health-care professionals.

Self-insured Employers

Self-insurance has become a popular option for more than 40% of medium and large corporations in the United States. Some analysts estimate that as many as 75% of the largest of the Fortune 500 companies are self-insured. Under this plan a company contributes a calculated rate into a special fund and then pays their employees' health-benefit claims from that fund. Some companies purchase traditional insurance for part of their claims and self-fund a fixed percentage.

FIGURE 7.5
PPO Trends

- Insurers and insurer-provider ventures at the forefront of PPO development and sponsorship
- Increased focus on documenting quality of care and cost-effectiveness
- Increased emphasis on prospective reimbursement, detailed utilization review (UR), data management, and benefits packages; decreased focus on discounting
- Thriving of regional PPO networks
- Employers demanding increased involvement in PPO plan design
- Development of specialty PPOs
    —occupational health
    —pharmacy
    —dental
    —other (possibly SLP/A)
- Hybrid PPOs/HMOs
    —merging of financing, underwriting, and delivery of care
    —blurring of differences between HMOs and PPOs; creation of new arrangements

This type of arrangement is known as a minimum-premium plan (MPP). Other corporations purchase only reinsurance or stop-loss insurance to cover the cost of catastrophic claims. Employers who assume all of the risk of paying employees' claims are self-funded.

The growth of self-insurance and self-funding has consequently diminished the market for conventional insurance plans but has expanded the market for insurance companies, managed-care companies, and third-party administrators who perform administrative, claims-processing, case-management, utilization review, and auditing services for self-insured employers. These employers are also channeling employees to alternative service delivery plans such as HMOs and PPOs.

According to the Employee Benefit Research Institute (1986), self-insurance plans offer more limited coverage than traditional plans for some services such as extended care, laboratory tests, mental health services, and alcoholism treatment. However, they typically provide enhanced coverage for primary-care services (e.g., routine physical exams, physician's office visits). Self-insured plans are exempt from state insurance regulation and mandated health benefits under the preemption allowed by the Employee Retirement Income Security Act of 1974. This exemption has raised a number of public-policy questions, and several bills have been introduced in Congress that would overturn the current law.

It is clear that self-insured-employer health-benefit plans are an important segment of private-sector health-care financing and service delivery. Rehabilitation professionals and other health-care providers will need to devise ways to educate employers about the value of covering their services. The provider-sponsored PPO will likely be an important option for health-care professionals to consider in reaching the self-insured-employer community.

The Uninsured

Most people in this country enjoy a full range of health benefits provided by employers or government programs. Others who can afford to do so purchase individual health insurance policies. About 37 million persons, however, have no insurance benefits. This number represents a 40% increase since 1980. Many of these persons are employed as seasonal or part-time workers, or are employees of small businesses. The remainder of this population is composed of children under 18, single mothers at home with young children, students, and other nonemployed persons. Part of the problem is the result of tightened eligibility requirements for Medicaid. Fewer than half the people whose incomes fall below the poverty line now meet Medicaid eligibility criteria. When the uninsured receive health-care services, they are usually unable to pay out-of-pocket.

Few persons can afford to pay the high cost of medical care without benefit of insurance. Consequently, hospitals provided about $9.5 billion of uncompensated and charity care last year. Cost-containment strategies have stripped away funding for charity care, so public and private health-care policymakers are

TABLE 7.2
A Comparison of Health-Care Financing/Delivery Models

Health Care Models	Who assumes risk?	Who pays providers and how?	Do incentives exist for the use of select providers?	What degree of control is exercised over provider practice patterns?
Traditional Insurance	Insurer	Insurer; fee for service	No	None
Traditional Insurance with PPO	Insurer	Insurer; prospectively negotiated, discounted fee for service	Limited	Strong, for PPO participating providers
Self-funded Organization	Employer or union trust fund	Employer or union trust fund; fee for services	No	None
Self-funded Organization with PPO	Employer or union trust fund	Employer or union trust fund; prospectively negotiated, discounted fee for services	Limited	Strong, for PPO participating providers
Self-funded Organization with EPO	Employer or union trust fund	Employer or union trust fund; prospectively negotiated, discounted fee for service	Extremely strong	Strong
Health Maintenance Organization (HMO)	HMO (employer/subscribing group pays premium)	HMO: physicians frequently paid on capitation basis	Extremely strong	Strong
Independent Practice Associations (IPA)	IPA (employer/subscribing group pays premium)	IPA: physician paid on capitation or fee-for-service basis	Extremely strong	Limited to strong

NOTE: From *The PPO Handbook* by S. Barger, D. Hillman, and H. Garland, 1985, Rockville, MD: Aspen Systems. Reprinted with permission of Aspen Publishers, Inc. Copyright 1985.

seeking ways to pay for health care for the uninsured and uninsurable, individuals who have a health problem for which no insurance company will provide benefits.

Congress has recently enacted legislation that requires states to extend Medicaid benefits to pregnant women and children under age five if they meet public assistance criteria. In addition, the Consolidated Omnibus Budget Reconciliation Act of 1985 (COBRA) prohibits hospitals from refusing emergency treatment to persons who have no health insurance. The law also requires employers to allow laid-off employees, employees' widows, divorced spouses, and dependent children to maintain group health benefits, paid for by the employee or spouse, for a specified period of time.

New legislation has been proposed that would require states to establish insurance risk pools. More formally known as comprehensive health insurance associations, risk pools are funds created by assessments on insurance companies, employers, and HMOs. In some cases, pools are partially funded by taxes. Uninsurable persons purchase coverage from the fund. Twelve states have already established risk pools; 13 states were considering legislation in early 1987. According to the Employee Benefit Research Institute (1986), premiums for pool coverage can often be higher than for individual or group health-insurance policies, so the problem of providing care for the growing uninsured population will probably not be solved in the near future.

■ SUMMARY

This section on private-sector health plans was intended to provide an overview of current financing and service delivery models and trends. Although we have discussed each component separately, it is increasingly difficult to delineate differences among plans as the private sector integrates and diversifies products and services. Table 7.2 was designed by Barger, Hillman, and Garland (1985) to help readers classify models according to risk, payment mechanisms, assessment of provider practice patterns, and patient utilization of services.

The private and public health-care sectors will continue to change rapidly throughout the next decade. At the same time, speech-language pathology and audiology services and practices are also evolving. Providing quality care and meeting the diverse needs of tomorrow's health-care system are among the most exciting challenges facing rehabilitation professionals today.

ACTIVITIES

1. Find out the details of your own health-insurance plan. Does it cover speech-language pathology and audiology services? (Check your benefits booklet. If you are covered by employee health benefits, ask your employee-benefits coordinator.) Are only certain communication disorders covered? May services be obtained from any speech-language pathologist or audiologist? Is a physician referral required? Are there dollar or time limits? Compare your coverage with that of colleagues. If you aren't satisfied with the coverage, what might you do to improve it?

2. Ask a Medicare beneficiary his/her opinion about the Medicare program. Perhaps the person can share some experiences with you about services, filing claims, Medigap policies, and other items.
3. What are the referral and reimbursement patterns in your clinic? What percentage of the clients is covered by a government or private health program for SLP/A services? What percent is paid out-of-pocket? Is your clinic an approved Blue Cross provider? Is the clinic Medicare certified? Perhaps the clinic director can meet with students to describe reimbursement trends and issues.
4. Investigate the availability of HMOs and PPOs in your area. Who sponsors them? Are local speech-language pathologists and audiologists involved? If so, how?

REFERENCES

Arnett, R., & Trapnell, G. (1984). Private health insurance: New measures of a complex and changing industry. *Health Care Financing Review, 6*(2), 31–42.

Barger, S., Hillman, D., & Garland, H. (1985). *The PPO handbook.* Rockville, MD: Aspen.

Blue Cross/Blue Shield of Maryland (1986, December 22). *Special memo: Gold standard coverage for outpatient speech-language pathology services and outpatient pretreatment certification.* Baltimore, MD: Blue Cross/Blue Shield of Maryland.

Chwat, S., & Gurland, G. (1984). National trends in third party reimbursement in speech-language pathology and audiology: Our professional crisis. *Asha, 26*(7), 27–32.

Cornett, B. (1987). Managed care: A primer. *Governmental Affairs Review, 8*(1), 38–42.

Cornett, B., & Chabon, S. (1986, November). Speech-language pathologists: Winners or losers in the health care revolution? Paper presented at the meeting of the American Speech-Language-Hearing Association, Detroit, MI.

Demkovich, L. (1986, January–February). Covering options through mandated benefits. *Business and Health, 3*(3), 27–29.

Downey, M., White, S., & Karr, S. (1984). *Health insurance manual for speech-language pathologists and audiologists.* Rockville, MD: American Speech-Language-Hearing Association.

Employee Benefit Research Institute. (1986, November). Features of employee health plans: Cost containment, plan funding, and coverage continuation. *Issue Brief No. 60.*

Farley, P. (1986, September). *Private health insurance in the U.S., National health care expenditures study data preview no. 23* (Publication No. PHS 86–3406). Washington, DC: U.S. Dept. of Health and Human Services, National Center for Health Services Research.

Fox, P., & Anderson, M. (1986, March). Hybrid HMOs, PPOs: The new focus. *Business and Health, 3*(4), 20–27.

Friedman, E. (1987, January 20). Medicaid's overload sparks a crisis. *Hospitals,* 50–54.

HIAA Consumer & Professional Relations Division (1986, April). *Report on consumer and professional relations: Speech-language pathology and audiology.* Washington, DC: Health Insurance Association of America.

White, S. (1986a). Third-party reimbursement. In R. McLauchlin (Ed.), *Speech-language pathology and audiology: Issues and management* (pp. 303–328). NY: Grune & Stratton.

————. (1986b). Licensure and third-party reimbursement. *Asha, 28*(6), 36.

Glossary

This glossary is divided into the following sections:

> Medicare and Medicaid Terms
> Health-Insurance-Industry Terms
> Alternative-Health-Care Terms
> Health-Care System Terms

It is intended as a "user-friendly" introduction to the confusing array of terms used in the health-care field. Although not exhaustive, the glossary is quite comprehensive and may serve as a quick reference for practicing professionals as well as graduate students in speech-language pathology.

A number of the terms are reproduced from *Health Care Reimbursement: A Glossary* (1983), reproduction with permission from

> Terry L. Schmidt Inc.
> Health Care Consultants
> 8950 Villa La Jolla Drive, Suite 1200
> La Jolla, CA 92037

MEDICARE AND MEDICAID TERMS

Assignment. A condition of payment for participants in Medicare Part B and some Blue Shield plans in which the provider agrees to accept the payment of the benefits plan as payment in full and no further charges are billed to the patient, even though the provider's usual fee may exceed the plan's payment.

Carrier. An organization that contracts with the Health Care Financing Administration to process claims and perform other services for the Medicare Part B program.

Comprehensive Outpatient Rehabilitation Facility (CORF). A Medicare provider type that is engaged in providing diagnostic, therapeutic, and rehabilitation services to outpatients. These services must include physician's services, physical therapy, and social or psychological services. Speech-language pathology may also be offered in a CORF.

Diagnosis Related Group (DRG). A system for classifying patients according to health-care resource consumption needs. Variables used for grouping patients include: age, principle diagnosis, surgical procedures, complications, and comorbid conditions. 467 DRGs are used as the basis of payment to hospitals under Medicare's Prospective Payment System.

Disabled. For purposes of enrollment in Medicare, individuals under age 65 are eligible to receive these benefits if they have been entitled to disability payments for not less than 24 months under the Social Security program or railroad retirement system.

Federal Employees Health Benefits Program (FEHBP). The group health insurance program for federal employees.

Health Care Financing Administration (HCFA). A principal operating component of the Department of Health and Human Services composed of organizational units with responsibilities related to the administration of Medicare, Medicaid, and supporting functions and services.

Home Health Agency (HHA).   A Medicare-certified agency that provides home health-care services (skilled nursing and rehabilitation services—physical therapy, occupational therapy, speech-language pathology, medical social services, home health aide) to eligible homebound patients who require skilled nursing, physical therapy, or speech-language pathology services on an intermittent basis.

Intermediary.   An organization selected by providers of health care that has entered into an agreement with the Department of Health and Human Services under Medicare's hospital insurance program (Part A) to process claims and perform other functions. Traditionally, intermediaries have been Blue Cross plans or insurance companies.

Intermediate Care Facility (ICF).   An institution licensed under state law to provide, on a regular basis, health care and services to individuals who do not require the degree of care and treatment that a hospital or a skilled nursing facility is designed to provide. Federal payment for ICF services is limited to Medicaid.

Major Diagnostic Categories (MDCs).   Grouping of *ICD-9-CM* codes into 23 broad classifications of diagnoses. Categories are defined considering anatomic classification, clinical management, number of patients included, and coverage of all codes without overlap. The 23 MDCs form the basis for the 467 DRGs upon which the Prospective Payment System is based.

Maximum Allowable Prevailing Charge (MAPC).   The list of upper limits that a carrier will allow in reimbursement of physicians' charges for services rendered to Medicare patients.

Medicaid.   Medicaid is a federally assisted program, operated by individual states, that provides medical benefits for eligible low-income persons (aged, blind, disabled, members of families with dependent children in which one is absent, disabled, or unemployed).

Medicare.   A program authorized by the Social Security Act of 1965, which assists in payment for medical and health services for persons age 65 and over, certain disabled persons, and those workers and their dependents who require kidney transplants or dialysis (end-stage renal disease). Income is not a consideration for participation in this program. *Part A* covers hospital, home health, hospice, and skilled-nursing facility (SNF) costs while *Part B* covers physician services and other outpatient services (for a monthly premium).

Medicare Provider Number.   The number assigned to a health-care provider by the Health Care Financing Administration, which administers the Medicare program.

Medicare Transmittal.   An information bulletin from HCFA sent to Medicare intermediaries and carriers that provides administrative direction, policy, or instructions necessary to administer the Medicare program.

Medicare Waiver of Liability.   A provision of Medicare law that protects the beneficiary from liability for payments to a provider for noncovered services or when services have been found not to be reasonable and necessary, and the beneficiary did not know or could not reasonably be expected to have known that the services were not covered.

Outliers.   Cases within each DRG that are extraordinarily costly to treat, relative to other cases, within a specific DRG (due to severity of illness, intensity of care required, complications, or need for excessive length of stay). Within specified guidelines, HCFA must provide additional payments for these cases to the provider.

Peer Review Organization (PRO).   A physician-sponsored organization whose purpose is to determine the appropriateness of care rendered to Medicare patients.

Prospective Payment/Reimbursement.   A method of paying hospitals or other health programs in which amounts/rates of payment are established in advance for the coming year and the programs are paid these fixed amounts, regardless of the costs they actually incur (see DRG).

Regulations. The set of rules promulgated by the executive branch of government to implement the legislation enacted by the legislative branch of government. Regulations have the force of law. In the federal government, legislation is enacted by Congress; then, the appropriate agency publishes a Notice of Intent (NOI) to develop regulations. Draft regulations are published in a Notice of Proposed Rule Making (NPRM) for public comment. After comments have been considered, Final Regulations are published. NOI, NPRM, and Final Regulations are published in the *Federal Register.*

Rehabilitation Agency (RA). A Medicare provider type that is an integrated multidisciplinary program designed to upgrade the physical functioning of the handicapped, disabled individual by bringing together a team of specialized rehabilitation personnel. RAs may be established by a speech-language pathologist or physical therapist who also includes social or vocational adjustment services as needed for the rehabilitation program.

Skilled-Nursing Facility (SNF). Under Medicare and Medicaid, an institution (or part of an institution) that has a transfer agreement with one or more participating hospitals and is primarily engaged in providing skilled-nursing care or rehabilitation services. The health care of each patient must be supervised by a physician.

Spend-down. As applied to the Medicaid program, the requirement that an individual's assets be reduced to a certain level to qualify for eligibility to participate in Medicaid. This term is usually applied to such requirements for persons who need long-term institutional care.

HEALTH-INSURANCE-INDUSTRY TERMS

Actuarial Tables. Statistical displays of calculations of life and/or health expectancy, used by actuaries in determining health-insurance premiums and annuities.

Adjudicate. To settle judicially a case of controversy. In reimbursement, claims controversies between beneficiaries, providers, or insurers are generally adjudicated through an insurer review board or other entity not involved in routine processing of claims.

All Payer System. Payment by all payers, private and insured, for hospital inpatient services on the basis of a prospective-payment methodology. The Federal Prospective Payment System (PPS) legislation requires the Secretary of the Department of Health and Human Services (DHHS) to study and report to Congress on the feasibility and desirability of expanding this methodology to all payers.

Beneficiary. A person who is eligible to receive, or is receiving, benefits from an insurance policy.

Benefit Package. A contractually defined set of health services, the cost of which is borne in full or in part by a health-insurance plan.

Blue Cross (BC). A nonprofit health-service prepayment organization providing coverage for hospital care and related services.

Blue Shield (BS). A nonprofit medical-service prepayment organization providing for medical care and related services.

Business Coalition. A group of employers (and sometimes representatives of labor unions, insurers, hospitals, and the medical community) in a given community or region whose purpose in forming an alliance is to promote health-care reform collectively.

A primary purpose of the coalition is usually to initiate or implement cost-containment efforts in the health-care industry. Activities of the coalition may include sponsorship of health, education and wellness programs; collection of local or regional health-care utilization, cost, and quality data; promoting alternative delivery systems; modifying employee-benefit programs; and negotiating discounts for health services provided to employee groups.

Cafeteria-Style Employee Benefits.   An employer benefit structure in which the employee may choose among an array of health and other benefits in a combination that best fits the needs of the employee. For example, an employee with children may want a large life-insurance policy and a dental plan, whereas a single person may opt for cash instead of certain benefits.

Claim.   A request to an insurer by an insured person or his assignee for payment of benefits under an insurance policy.

Claims Review.   Review of claims by governments, medical foundations, insurers, or others responsible for payment to determine liability and amount of payment. This review may include determination of the eligibility of the claimant or beneficiary; or the eligibility of the provider of the benefit; that the benefit for which payment is claimed is covered; that the benefit is not payable under another policy; and that the benefit was necessary and of reasonable cost and quality.

Coinsurance.   Established percentages indicating the portion of covered expenses, beyond the deductible, to be paid under the coverage and the portion to be borne by the subscriber (patient).

Commercial Insurance.   Private health insurance sold or underwritten by a for-profit insurance company.

Community Rating.   A method of establishing premiums for health insurance in which the premium is based on the average cost of actual or anticipated health care used by all subscribers in a specific geographic area or industry, which does not vary for different groups or subgroups or subscribers, or with such variables as the group's claims experience, age, sex, or health status.

Coordination of Benefits (COB).   Integration of benefits payable under more than one health-insurance plan, so that benefits from all sources do not exceed 100% of the total allowable medical expenses.

Copayment.   A type of health-care cost sharing whereby the insured or covered person pays a fixed amount per unit of medical service or unit of time and the insurer pays the rest of the cost.

Cost Shifting.   The practice of charging private-paying patients and those covered by commercial insurance for costs not allowed by Blue Cross, Medicare, and Medicaid.

Deductible.   A fixed amount that an insured person must expend on medical services before the insurer will pay for the services.

Eligibility.   The status of a person in regard to an insurance contract or program. A person having eligibility is entitled to receive benefits under the contract or program.

Exclusions.   Specific hazards, perils, or conditions listed in an insurance or medical-care-coverage policy for which the policy will not provide benefit payments. Common exclusions include preexisting conditions such as heart disease, diabetes, or a pregnancy begun before the policy was in effect.

Experience Rating.   A method of establishing premiums for health insurance in which the premium is based on the average cost of actual or anticipated health care used by various groups or anticipated health care used by various groups and subgroups of subscribers. It is the most common method of establishing premiums for health insurance in private programs.

Group Insurance.   Any insurance plan in which a number of employees of an employer (and their dependents), or members of a similar homogeneous group, are insured under a single policy, issued to their employer or the group with individual certificates of insurance given to each insured individual.

Health Insurance.   Insurance against loss by disease or accidental bodily injury. Such insurance usually covers some of the medical costs of treating the disease or injury, may cover other losses associated with them, and may be either individual or group insurance.

Indemnity Benefits.   The provision of benefits on the basis of a set dollar allowance for covered services. The indemnity insurance contract usually defines the maximum amounts that will be paid for the covered services.

Insurance Policy.   A written contract of insurance. One party agrees to reimburse another for loss to a person or thing caused by designated contingencies. Insurance is a formal social device for reducing the risk of losses to individuals by spreading the risk over groups.

Major Medical.   The insurance program that allows payment of a major portion or reasonable and customary charges for covered services to the extent not covered by basic health insurance, and is designed to offset the heavy medical expenses resulting from catastrophic or prolonged illness or injuries.

Medical Necessity.   A determination by a health insurer of a patient's need for medical services in the setting provided, or in accordance with a health-insurance policy.

Medicare Supplemental Policy.   Often called Medigap, a health-insurance policy offered to Medicare beneficiaries by insurance companies that provides payment for services/items not covered by Medicare.

Out-of-Pocket Expenses.   Those expenses paid directly by patients to providers, either because they are not covered by insurance, or as part of deductible and copayment provisions.

Preexisting Condition.   An injury, disease, or physical condition that existed prior to the issuance of a health-insurance policy and usually results in exclusion from coverage under the policy for treatment related to those conditions.

Premium.   The amount of money that is paid by an insured person or policyholder to an insurer or third party for health-insurance coverage under a health-insurance policy.

Prudent Buyer.   A purchaser of goods or services who seeks to obtain the greatest quantity and highest quality of services for the least cost.

Reinsurance.   An insurance company for insurance companies—the practice of one insurance company purchasing insurance from a second company for the purpose of protecting itself against part or all of the losses it might incur in the process of honoring policyholders' claims.

Relative Value Scale (RVS).   A system for determining the value of health professionals' services by units. Services of the same type are compared according to a determined unit value. Conversion factors are applied to relative value units to arrive at fee schedules.

Reserve.   A sum set aside by an insurance company to guarantee the fulfillment of commitments for future claims.

Risk.   A chance of loss. In the insurance field, risk is determined by actuarial tables. The insurance company bases its policies and premiums on the probability that illnesses, accidents, or deaths will occur in certain populations.

Self-insurance.   The practice of an individual, group, employer, or organization assuming responsibility for losses such as medical expenses rather than paying premiums to an insurance company.

Self-pay.   The practice of paying for health-care services out of pocket. Individuals who self-pay either have no insurance benefits or are paying for services, procedures, or products not covered by their insurance plans.

Service Benefit.   Health benefits provided in the form of hospital or medical care. Service benefits are offered by the Blue Cross/Blue Shield plans. Other insurance plans make monetary payments to subscribers or policyholders to offset losses incurred in paying for health-care services (indemnity benefits).

Third-Party Administrator (TPA).   An entity that contracts with insurers or providers to process health-insurance claims. May also perform utilization review but does not establish policies for insurance companies.

Third-Party Payer.   An organization that pays or insures health or medical expenses on behalf of beneficiaries or recipients. The three parties in this process include the individual receiving the service (first party), the individual or institution providing the service (second party), and the organization paying for services (third party).

Usual, Customary, and Reasonable (UCR).   A method of payment that allows the physician's usual charge unless it exceeds the customary allowance, or the amount customarily charged by other physicians in a geographic area, unless it is determined to be a reasonable amount for the services rendered.

Waiting Period.   The period of time an individual must wait either to become eligible for insurance coverage or to become eligible for a given benefit after overall coverage has begun.

ALTERNATIVE-HEALTH-CARE TERMS

Alternative Delivery System (ADS).   A way of organizing health care based on the premise that an alternative is needed to the traditional solo practice, fee-for-service model. In ADS plans, services are offered in ways designed to improve accessibility, continuity, and quality of care while containing or reducing costs.

Capitation.   A method of health-care payment in which a uniform per capita fee or premium is paid on a fixed basis, independent of the number or type of services received during that period.

Competitive Medical Plan (CMP).   A health-care plan that provides a range of inpatient and outpatient services to an enrolled population for a periodic fee. The CMP assumes financial risk for providing those services and meets certain requirements to assure financial solvency. Although CMPs must provide the same services to Medicare beneficiaries as federally qualified HMOs, for non-Medicare enrollees CMPs may set premium rates on the basis of the health experience of specific groups (experience rating), be a line of business and not a separate legal entity, and charge enrollees copayments and deductibles with no restrictions. There is no requirement for open enrollment periods or for offering more expensive care such as mental health and substance-abuse services and home health. Although employers with more than 25 employees must offer a federally qualified HMO as a health-benefit plan option, they are not required to offer a CMP.

Enrollee.   One who enrolls in a prepaid health program for health services. The terms of enrollment are understood to mean that the health-delivery program provides, or contracts for, an agreed upon list of health services for a given period of time in return for a fixed payment or premium.

Gatekeeper.   A primary-care physician, physician specialist, or other health-care professional (often a registered nurse) who authorizes and monitors health-care services covered by a health-care plan for a defined patient population.

Health Maintenance Organization (HMO).   Any organization that, through an organized system of health care, provides or assures the delivery of an agreed upon set of comprehensive health-maintenance and treatment services for an enrolled group of persons under a prepaid fixed sum or capitation arrangement.

Independent Practice Association (IPA).   A health maintenance organization delivery mode in which an association made up of individual private practitioners contracts to provide services to HMO enrollees. The HMO usually pays the IPA on a prepaid capitation basis to provide a defined package of services to its enrollees. However, the IPA may pay its members on a fee-for-service basis.

Preferred Provider Organization (PPO).   An insurance arrangement whereby insurers contract with providers for certain services based on a fee schedule. Plan members are then encouraged to use the "preferred" provider panel when seeking medical and related services. If the plan member chooses providers outside the panel, he/she must then pay the difference between those charges and the approved fee schedule.

Prepaid Group Practice (PPGP).   A health plan in which a health organization (or a formal association of three or more physicians) contracts to provide a specified set of services to the health-plan enrollees in return for a fixed periodic payment per enrollee (also known as a group-model HMO).

HEALTH-CARE SYSTEM TERMS

Accreditation.   The process by which an agency or organization evaluates and recognizes a program of study or an institution as meeting certain predetermined standards. Accreditation is usually given by a private organization created for the purpose of assuring the public of the quality of the accredited program.

Acute Care.   Care for victims of acute disease or injury or acute exacerbation of chronic disease. Acute-care provision requires availability of a comprehensive array of services and skills, and concentrated continuous care.

Ambulatory Care.   Delivery of health-care services on an outpatient basis.

Ambulatory Surgery.   Surgery that does not require inpatient admission to a hospital.

Ancillary Care.   Health services other than physician or nursing services or hospital room and board; may include hospital, x-ray, drug, laboratory, and therapy services.

Audit.   A systematic review of provider records to determine whether service claimed has been provided and to verify the nature of the service and adherence to program policies and procedures.

Case Mix.   The diagnosis-specific makeup of a health program's work load. Case mix directly influences the length of stay, intensity, cost, and scope of the services provided by a hospital or other health program.

Commission on Accreditation of Rehabilitation Facilities (CARF).   A national private, nonprofit organization that sets standards and accredits facilities providing services to physically and developmentally disabled persons.

Diagnostic and Statistical Manual of Mental Disorders (DSM).   A publication of the American Psychiatric Association that defines mental disorders and describes diagnostic criteria and approaches to evaluation of persons with mental disorders (classifies many communication disorders).

Discharge. Formal release of a patient from the hospital or other health-care program.

Durable Medical Equipment (DME). Equipment that can stand repeated use, is primarily and customarily used to serve a medical purpose, generally is not useful to a person in the absence of illness or injury, and is appropriate for use in the home.

Fee-for-service. A method of paying for medical care in which patients are charged a specified amount for each service provided.

Home Health Care. Health services rendered to an individual as needed in the home. Such services are provided to aged, disabled, sick, or convalescent individuals who do not need hospital care. The services may be provided by a visiting-nurse association, home health agency, hospital, or other organized community group. Under Medicare, services must be provided by a Medicare-certified home health agency.

Hospice. A program that provides palliative and supportive care for terminally ill patients and their families, either directly or on a consulting basis with the patient's physician or another community agency. Emphasis is placed on symptom control, a preparation for and support before and after death.

Inpatient Day. A day of care furnished any inpatient except a newborn occupying a nursery bassinet and excluding days of care in an intensive-care unit or skilled-nursing facility (SNF).

International Classification of Diseases, 9th Edition, Clinical Modifications (ICD-9-CM). A system developed for classifying diseases and operations, and for indexing of hospital records. Diseases are grouped according to the problems they present. The coding system was developed for the clinical management of patient problems and the generating of indicators of health status and health statistics.

Joint Commission on Accreditation of Healthcare Organizations (JCAHO). A private nonprofit organization dedicated to promoting quality health care through a voluntary accreditation process. JCAHO is governed by a 22-member Board of Commissioners. More than 45 health-care organizations have representatives on JCAHO advisory committees. JCAHO publishes standards for hospitals, long-term-care, ambulatory-care, hospice, and psychiatric and substance-abuse facilities.

Length of Stay (LOS). The length of an inpatient's stay in a hospital reported as the number of days spent in a facility per admission or discharge.

Long-Term Care (LTC). Includes all services, both institutional and noninstitutional, that are required by all people with chronic health conditions. Such conditions may be experienced at any age as recurrent or persistent symptoms, illness, disability, or impairment of a physical or mental nature.

Medical Case Management. A system of assessment, treatment planning, and follow-up that seeks to provide coordinated, comprehensive health-care services for the patient while minimizing costs to the payer. A case manager (usually a registered nurse or other rehabilitation specialist) is responsible for coordinating service delivery and payment. Medical-case-management services are initiated primarily for high-cost cases that will require long-term and/or intensive medical and rehabilitation services.

Medical Record. A written document that contains sufficient information to identify the patient clearly, to justify the diagnosis and treatment, and to document the results accurately.

Medical Rehabilitation. Professional and technical services that promote maximum functional independence in patients who have physical disabilities. Treatments and procedures are designed to minimize impairments, restore lost or reduced functional capacities, and facilitate adaptation to permanent disability.

Medical Review.   Review by a team of health-care professionals of the condition and need for care. Medical review differs from utilization review in that it requires evaluation of each individual patient and an analysis of the appropriateness of treatment rendered in a specific institution (utilization review is often done on a sample basis and focuses on certain procedures, conditions, or lengths of stay).

Outpatient Services.   Medical and other services provided by a hospital, other facility, or supplier to persons who are not inpatients.

Overutilization.   Unnecessary or excessive rendering of services by providers, or demand for services by patients.

Peer Review.   Evaluation by physicians or other health-care professionals of the effectiveness and efficiency of services ordered or performed by other professionals whose work is being reviewed (peers).

Prior Authorization.   Requirement imposed by a third party, under some systems of utilization review, that a provider must justify before a peer-review committee, insurance representative, or state agent the need for delivering a particular service to a patient, before providing the service, in order to receive reimbursement (also called precertification).

Provider.   An individual or institution that provides medical care (physician and other health-care professionals, hospitals, skilled-nursing facilities, rehabilitation centers, rehabilitation agencies, clinics, public health agencies).

Quality Assurance (QA).   Activities and programs intended to assure the quality of care delivered in a defined setting. These activities include identification of deficiencies in care, analysis of deficiencies, and development of a plan of action to remedy problems identified.

Tertiary Care.   Subspecialty care usually requiring facilities of a university-affiliated or teaching hospital that has extensive diagnostic and treatment capabilities.

Utilization.   Patterns or rates of use of a type of service.

Utilization Review (UR).   Evaluation of the necessity, appropriateness, and efficiency of the use of medical services, procedures, and facilities. This review may be completed by in-house coordinators and/or committees, public agencies, or Peer Review Organizations (PROs).

Vendor.   A provider, institution, agency, organization, or individual practitioner who provides health or medical services or equipment.

CHAPTER EIGHT

*Evaluating the Quality of Care**

INTRODUCTION

A new—or perhaps renewed—concern for quality and value has permeated our society. We have become demanding consumers. Our food, clothing, and cars have been subject to vigorous scrutiny as we seek to purchase quality goods at reasonable prices. America's automobile industry has faced probably the toughest challenge to the quality of its products with the advent of the high-performance and low-repair-rate cars associated with Japanese automakers. Most consumers think of the phrase ''made in Japan'' as a mark of high quality, not only for automobiles but for televisions, radios, computers, stereos, and many other products. Consequently, American industry has begun to focus again on producing quality goods at reasonable prices. One of our ''big three'' automakers advertises that ''Quality Is Job One'' and emphasizes its warranty as a selling point.

We Americans are also concerned about spending ''quality time'' with our families and friends, being efficient students or employees, using our leisure time to keep mentally and physically fit, and improving the quality of government services, public education, and health care. The public education system has

*The authors wish to acknowledge Dr. Carol Frattali for her numerous contributions to the content and format of this chapter.

recently responded to allegations that America's children have been receiving a less-than-quality education by focusing on a return to "basic" courses like math, reading, and science and less on social issues. In addition, national teacher-competency standards and examinations are being developed, as well as mechanisms for evaluating teachers' job performance based on such indicators as students' test scores, supervisors' observations, and other subjective and objective data. Finally, colleges and universities are attempting to develop ways to attract high-quality young adults to the teaching profession to reverse the trend toward low college-achievement test scores among persons selecting education as a major.

During the past few years, the health-care system has been occupied primarily with attempting to reduce or contain the escalating costs of patient care, especially in hospitals. Although quality has always been an important concern, cost issues have compelled health-care professionals to demonstrate the value of health-care services, that is, the benefits of care in relation to the cost incurred. As a result, members of the health-care community have been subject to increasing scrutiny by being asked to define quality, identify appropriate types and levels of care, devise ways to measure the quality of health-care services, and provide convincing utilization data.

This chapter presents an overview of information about current developments in the health-care system related to defining, evaluating, and attempting to assure the provision of quality health care. In part 1 we discuss the general health-care system and its mechanisms for assessing quality and appropriate utilization of resources. In part 2 we focus on quality of care in speech-language pathology and audiology.

QUALITY AND THE HEALTH-CARE SYSTEM

In Search of a Definition of Quality

Everyone seems to agree on the need to provide quality health care, but there is no consensus on how to define it. Avedis Donabedian, one of the major proponents of the quality movement, says that quality care is "that kind of care which is expected to maximize an inclusive measure of patient welfare, after one has taken account of the balance of expected gains and loses that attend the process of care in all its parts" (1980, p. 5). According to Donabedian, the attributes of quality care include accessibility, acceptability, continuity, and coordination of health-care services; patient and practitioner satisfaction; prevention and early detection of disease or illness; and efficiency, effectiveness, and uniformity of services.

During its 1986 annual meeting, the American Medical Association issued the statement that high-quality care should (1) produce optimal improvement in a patient's physical and emotional status as quickly as possible; (2) emphasize the promotion of health and the prevention and early detection of disease; (3) involve the patient in decision making; (4) be based on accepted principles of medical science; (5) include sensitivity to patients' stress and anxiety associated with illness; (6) make efficient use of technological and professional resources; and (7) be sufficiently documented to facilitate continuity of care and peer review.

Another definition is provided by the U.S. Congress's Office of Technology Assessment (1986): quality of care is defined as "the degree to which actions taken or not taken maximize the probability of beneficial health outcomes and minimize risk and other untoward outcomes, given the existing state of medical science and art" (p. xii). Therefore, the definition of quality evolves with the state of the art and science of health care. Definitions will also change as we develop better ways to evaluate individual patient care and health programs. Definitions of quality also depend upon one's perspective—practitioner, policymaker, insurer, employer, or patient—and may include emphasis on technical or interpersonal aspects of care as well as concern for credentials, conformance to standards, cost-effective and efficient utilization of services, and amenities of care. Regardless of which definition or combination of definitions one accepts, the assessment of quality, says Donabedian (1980, p. ix), may be the most "central issue of all" in health care today. Quality, he continues, is a property that health care has in varying degrees. Our ability to "assure" quality depends upon our capability to evaluate accurately all aspects of the health-care process. This capability is rapidly increasing as the health-care community focuses on quality assessment and program evaluation activities.

Quality Assessment: Structure, Process, and Outcome

Judgments about the quality of health care are based upon what we know about the relationship between the health-care process and its consequences to individual and societal health and welfare, in accordance with the value we place on health care in our society (Donabedian, 1980). In the past, credentialing of health-care professionals and accrediting of facilities were the primary means of determining that quality services were being provided by practitioners and hospitals or other health-care programs. Assessments of quality thus focused on structural considerations; that is, the human, physical, and financial resources, or what Donabedian calls the "environment of care." These resources include the physical plant; supplies, equipment, and technology; staff size, training, experience, and qualifications; and administrative organization, policies, and procedures. Although structure can increase or decrease the probability of good performance, structure as a means of assessing quality poses some difficulties. According to Donabedian, the relative stability of the elements of structure makes it unsuitable for continuous monitoring activities. Also, we do not have enough empirical evidence regarding the influence of structural components on the quality of patient care to make judgments about quality based solely on structural considerations. Structure is, however, important in planning, designing, and implementing systems for the provision of health-care services and serves as a constant in the total patient-care-assessment process.

More recently, quality assessment procedures have focused on the entire process of care, including diagnosis, treatment, discharge planning, and follow-up or aftercare. Process considerations also include evaluation of mechanisms for documenting care, appropriate supervision of personnel, and patient-practitioner and intraprofessional relationships. Determinations are made about the accessibility and availability of patient care, continuity of treatment, coordination of services among practitioners, and efficiency of services. The growing market for case-management services is based upon the premise that a central figure, the case manager, is needed to assure the provision of efficient, coordinated service among patient-care team members. Case-management programs and companies market their services to employers and insurers by promising to reduce health-care costs through improvements in the overall process of patient care.

Quality assessment based on process assumes that the practitioner's adherence to standards is the key to quality patient care. Standards of care refer to accepted procedures that signify criteria for judging the appropriateness or adequacy of care. These standards, or established levels of performance, are determined by the state of the art and science of practice at the time of application. Process evaluations, then, determine the degree to which patient management conforms to the standards and expectations of accepted professional practice for a given profession. The major weakness of using process criteria alone to assess quality is that there is little scientific basis for most patient-care procedures. Furthermore, research has yet to show the relationships between particular elements of care and specific patient health outcomes (Donabedian, 1980).

The assessment of patient outcomes as the result of treatment is the current focus of debate and study in the health-care community. *Outcome* refers to the result of patient care—"the final evidence of whether care has been good, bad or indifferent" (Donabedian, 1969, p. 2). The emphasis on patient outcomes is consistent with the growing demand for evidence of cost-effectiveness and efficiency in the health-care system. Health-care professionals are being asked to document patients' need for services provided by demonstrating the specific impact of treatment on their health status. Practitioners must be able to identify the procedures that are associated with positive outcomes, those that may have a negative impact on health status, and those that appear to have a minimal influence on outcome. According to Donabedian (1980), the key to outcome assessment is that the patient's health status must be attributable to the actual care received and not to variables unrelated to the process of care.

In an effort to begin addressing these concerns, health-care practitioners and researchers are developing patient health-status and functional assessment measures designed to determine the relationship between treatment (process) and patient outcomes. Computer programs such as APACHE II and MedisGroups have been developed to classify patients according to severity of illness, thereby enabling practitioners to account for complicating factors in assessing the effectiveness of patient care. APACHE II, an acronym for "acute physiology and chronic health evaluation," uses 12 physiologic variables to create a "risk severity score." APACHE is used to monitor utilization and quality of care in intensive-care units.

MedisGroups or Medical Illness Severity Index, a software program that measures admission severity, patient complication rates, and outcomes, is designed to help providers determine appropriate and cost-efficient care. The program validates clinical procedures by comparing provider practice patterns with national clinical norms and standards.

The Joint Commission on Accreditation of Healthcare Organizations (JCAHO)—known until fall 1987 as the Joint Commission on Accreditation of Hospitals (JCAH)—is setting the pace in quality assessment by refocusing the health-facility accreditation process from a structure-process evaluation, or assessment of the capability of facilities and programs to provide quality care, to an assessment of whether quality health care is actually delivered. JCAHO will be developing indicators of care and criteria for appropriate care. The commission will be working with health-care professional associations in developing indicators, criteria, and functional assessment measures. In the initial stages of the new accreditation process, JCAHO will focus on the "avoidable outcomes" associated with high-volume, high-risk services such as obstetrics and anethesia. By 1990, JCAHO hopes to have in place a full set of clinical outcome measures incorporated into its standards for accreditation in all programs: hospitals, long-term-care facilities, ambulatory health-care programs, psychiatric facilities, hospices, community mental health services, alcohol and drug abuse programs, mental retardation/developmental disability (MR/DD) programs, and home-care services.

Quality assessment protocols, whether focused on structure, process, outcome, or a combination of factors, are based on explicit and/or implicit review criteria. Explicit criteria compare actual services or results with specific written indicators and must be stated in objective terms so that the possibility of individual interpretation is minimized and the care being evaluated can be specifically documented. These criteria must also conform with generally accepted standards of care in a given health-care profession. Ideally, explicit criteria are based on empirically derived standards of care. In contrast, implicit review criteria consist of professional judgments about quality care in which the evaluator makes decisions about quality of care based upon his or her education, experience, and expertise (Frattali, 1986; Haffner, Jonas, & Pollack, 1984). Adair and Griffin (1979) assert that effective reviews use both explicit and implicit criteria. Explicit criteria serve as screening mechanisms or critical indicators of quality care. Documented patient care that does not conform with the explicit criteria is then reviewed by peer professionals who make final judgments about whether discrepancies represent deficiencies or acceptable exceptions to the recognized standards of care.

Review criteria are applied to a variety of data sources. The most common data source is the patient record. Other sources include surveys, questionnaires, interviews, and direct observation. The computer is rapidly replacing the handwritten patient record as the preferred data source. Automation permits evaluators to study productivity, practice patterns, and patient outcomes for individuals and groups of practitioners, as well as resource-utilization patterns among service units or departments. Using these data sources, assessments may be conducted prospectively, concurrently, or retrospectively. Until recently, most assessments were retrospective studies, or record audits, conducted after services were rendered. The intention was to identify patterns of care so that any needed improvements could be made for future patients. Concurrent reviews are conducted during patient treatment and are often used to determine the need for continued stays in a health facility or treatment program. They are also used to assess appropriateness of procedures used in treatment as they occur. Prospective reviews use established admission criteria to determine the need for patient admissions to hospitals or other health-care programs (Arnold & Leonard, 1987). The need for ancillary and/or rehabilitation services may also be determined as part of both prospective and concurrent review systems.

Retrospective, concurrent, and prospective quality reviews all have merit for different types of assessments. The purpose and objectives of the assessment will largely dictate the temporal aspects of the review. According to Frattali (1986),

> The assessment of outcome is almost always retrospective since outcomes are often thought of as phenomena that occur subsequent to care. However, a study can be attempted so early that outcomes are not yet fully known or so late that the results have lost some of their usefulness. Retrospective studies do have the advantage of preventing bias in treatment practices if practitioners under concurrent or prospective study were aware of the study objectives. In many instances, retrospective rather than concurrent studies allow investigation of a larger defined population since they can span years of treatment. The major limitation of retrospective studies is the possible occurrence of incomplete documentation of care. Consequently, quality assessment using this method of study can be both inconclusive and invalid. (p. 6)

As the health-care system moves from retrospective reviews based on structural considerations to concurrent and prospective reviews based on process and outcome criteria, health-care professionals must develop valid and reliable measures that lend themselves to ongoing assessments of the patient-care process as well as the expected and actual outcomes of treatment. In order to attribute changes in patient health status to treatment, Donabedian (1980) advises that process and outcome elements must be studied simultaneously, when possible.

At this stage in the development of quality-assessment measures, the emphasis is on developing stronger criteria so that the focus of patient-care evaluation can gradually broaden to identify levels of quality care—satisfactory, good, and excellent. It is hoped that someday patient-care evaluation studies will be able to identify top-quality care, or care that "yields the greatest expected improvement in health status, health being defined very broadly to include physical, physiological, and psychological dimensions" (Donabedian, Wheeler, & Wyszewianski, 1984, p. 66).

Program Evaluation

Assessments of the quality of patient care and program evaluation are closely related in that both processes may involve the same data sources, categories or levels of evaluation, and study designs. The two assessments differ, however, in purpose and scope. Patient-care evaluations compare the objectives of individual patient care with actual treatments provided and results obtained. The purpose of program evaluation is to determine how well a program or a specific component of a program attains its goals. For example, the overall objective of a community speech-language-hearing clinic may be to meet the needs of the communicatively handicapped in a particular community. An evaluation of the program would help determine whether community needs are indeed being met. In addition to assessing the quality of patient care, a program evaluation may also review the clinic's administrative policies and procedures; operational functions such as marketing, communications, billing practices, and scheduling; and clinic staff development programs.

In determining whether a program is fulfilling its objectives, evaluators consider the reasonableness of program objectives as well as program costs in relation to benefits received. Additionally, program evaluation studies also attempt to determine reasons for specific program successes and failures, define strategies for increasing program effectiveness, and delineate those principles and activities that underlie successful programs. Results of program-evaluation studies should provide helpful information for program planning, development, and operation. The overall intention is to increase the effectiveness of program administration.

The evaluation process involves four basic steps: (1) delineation of program goals, (2) transfer of goals into measurable indicators of goal achievement, (3) data collection on the indicators, and (4) comparison of the data with program objectives. Program-evaluation studies may use a variety of data sources and evaluation designs. The stringency of the design should match the development of the program. Common evaluation designs include the one-time case study, static group comparison, pretest/post-test, and pretest/post-test with control group.

In the one-time case-study technique, observations and measurements are made after an individual's exposure to the program or treatment. Pretest/post-test designs obtain baseline measures before program participation and repeat the measures after program completion. The static group comparison study is sometimes difficult to undertake in health care. The performance of a treatment or participant group is compared with a group that does not receive treatment or participate in a program. In the pretest/post-test with control group design, subjects are randomly assigned to experimental or control groups. Observations or measurements are taken before and after program participation in both groups, even though only the experimental group participated. The one-time case-study approach is often considered the weakest form of evaluation research, whereas the pretest/post-test with control group design is considered to be the strongest in permitting evaluators to conclude that results can be attributed to the program.

The levels or categories of program evaluation are roughly analogous to the structure-process-outcome focus of quality assessment. These categories include effort, performance, adequacy of performance, efficiency, and process (Suchman, 1967). *Effort* refers to the energy expended by providers and may be determined by indicators such as number of clinic visits, treatment sessions, or materials purchased. *Performance* measures the results of the effort expended. For example, how many persons were actually rehabilitated in a drug treatment program? How many children were identified, evaluated, and successfully placed in early special education programs as a result of "Child Find" efforts? How many persons lost weight as a result of participating in a weight-reduction clinic? *Adequacy-of-performance* criteria involve the degree to which a program meets the total need. Measurement of adequacy often depends only on estimates of need for programs in a community, because accurate prevalence and incidence data are often not available. *Efficiency* refers to the ability of a program to accomplish its objectives in a timely manner and attempts to answer questions relative to the feasibility of using alternative methods or less costly resources. According to Suchman (1967), "The criteria of efficiency are coming more and more to dominate the evaluation picture" (p. 64). As health and education systems attempt to streamline programs and cut costs, policymakers and evaluators are focusing on how to accomplish objectives in less time, or with fewer or alternative human, financial, or material resources. Finally, the *process* category of program evaluation is what Suchman calls the "making sense" level. An analysis of process is intended to identify specific program components that contribute to or detract from program performance, and to establish a correlation between program activities and results obtained. Figure 8.1 provides an outline of the program-evaluation process.

According to Affeldt and Walczak (1984), the problems in patient care identified through program evaluation may be addressed through mechanisms established by a facility's quality-assurance program. That component of program evaluation may be considered part of the overall quality-assurance process. Other components, including operational and administrative functions, provide management with a system of accountability and function as a management tool. The program-evaluation process can also be used to evaluate the quality-assurance program itself. In the next section we define the objectives, components, and activities of quality-assurance programs.

Quality Assurance Programs

Quality Assurance

Quality assessment comprises the measurement phase of the quality-assurance process. The quality assurance program itself is an "action plan" designed to develop and implement solutions to problems (Adair & Griffin, 1979). Pena et al. (1984) define quality assurance as "the process that sets the standards for performance, provides information about the achievement of those standards, and monitors whether improvement has taken place and whether the standards are being met" (p. xiv). The quality assurance program model consists of an ongoing series of activities including:

1. Problem identification
2. Problem assessment/evaluation

FIGURE 8.1
Program Evaluation

Program Objectives: Program Results
Categories of Evaluation
Effort
Performance (Outcome)
Adequacy of Program
(in relation to community need)
Efficiency
Process
Data Sources
Interviews   Observation
(professionals/patients)
Patient Records
(individual)
Patient/Agency Records
(Aggregate)
Evaluation Designs
One-Time Case Study
Static Group Comparison
Pretest, Post-test
Pretest, Post-test Control Groups
Phases of Evaluation*
Delineate Program Goals
Specify Measurable Indicators of Goal Achievement
Collect Data
Compare Data with Program Objectives

*These phases denote steps in an outcome-focused study. A process-oriented study focuses on how staff members attempt to meet program objectives.

NOTE: Adapted from Handout for Graduate Course in Evaluation Research, by E. M. Ricci, Winter 1985, Pittsburgh, PA: Graduate School of Public Health, University of Pittsburgh. Used with permission.

3. Report of findings
4. Corrective action to eliminate or reduce deficiencies
5. Follow-up studies to assess effectiveness of corrective action
6. Continuous monitoring of all activities related to evaluation and patient care

This process may be thought of as a loop because the program provides for continuous repetition and refinement of activities. The Quality Assurance (QA) Loop is illustrated in Figure 8.2.

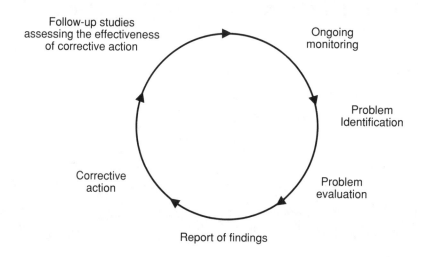

FIGURE 8.2
Quality Assurance Loop

NOTE: From *Handbook for Conduct of Medical Care Evaluation Studies* by Health Standards and Quality Bureau, Health Care Financing Administration, Department of Health, Education and Welfare, 1978, Washington, DC: U.S. Government Printing Office.

In its standards for hospital accreditation, the Joint Commission on Accreditation of Healthcare Organizations requires "an ongoing quality assurance program designed to objectively and systematically monitor and evaluate the quality and appropriateness of patient care, pursue opportunities to improve patient care, and resolve identified problems" (Joint Commission on Accreditation of Hospitals, 1986, p. 215). All services provided by professional staff as well as hospital departments and units are subject to quality assurance activities. In addition, infection-control, utilization review, and risk-management activities are considered part of the hospital's overall quality assurance program. In the evaluation process the quality assurance program must use "objective criteria that reflect current knowledge and clinical experience" (American Hospital Association, 1986, p. 217). For a description of evaluation criteria, temporal aspects, and types of assessments, the reader is directed to the discussion of quality assessment in this chapter.

The inclusion of utilization review activities in quality assurance programs is based on the premise that appropriate allocation and utilization of resources are indicators of quality health care. Donabedian (1980) contends that "quality costs money" but also maintains that quality is best served when unneccessary or excessive services are eliminated and necessary services are delivered more efficiently. Kearns (1984) describes the interaction between utilization review (UR) and quality assurance as follows:

> Quality assurance was conceived to enhance UR, but in reality it envelops UR along with program evaluation, auditing, credentialing, continuing medical education, monitoring and risk management. It envelops and at the same time is composed of the preceding tools, for without them there would be no efficiency, no effectiveness, and no quality. (p. 239)

Utilization Review

The goal of utilization review (UR) is the melding of quality with cost-management principles. Its purpose is to ensure the appropriate allocation of resources in providing patient care. Essentially, utilization review is a system for evaluating the necessity, appropriateness, and efficiency of health-care services delivered in both inpatient and outpatient settings. In its standards for accreditation, the Joint Commission on Accreditation of Healthcare Organizations requires that the health facility's UR program address overutilization, underutilization, and inefficient scheduling of resources (Joint Commission on Accreditation of Hospitals, 1986).

Utilization review activities can encompass every aspect of patient care, from a determination of the need for a patient's admission to a hospital to an examination of appropriateness of a discharge plan to study of suspected under-utilization of outpatient rehabilitation services. Reviews may be conducted prior to service delivery (prospectively), during a hospital stay or treatment period (concurrently), or after patient discharge (retrospectively) and most often involve review of patient records, although results of quality assurance studies, reimbursement agency utilization reports, practitioner profile analyses, and other documents are also used. Prospective reviews for hospitals base admission decisions on criteria established by the hospital or external agency for "medical necessity," appropriateness, and length-of-stay norms for a hospital's level of care. Concurrent reviews determine the need for continued stays and appropriateness of services and procedures provided to patients. Retrospective reviews are conducted primarily to identify patterns of care for analysis. The results are then incorporated into the quality assurance program for problem identification, resolution, and follow-up.

Utilization review programs were initially developed in response to federal government mandates. Since its inception, the Medicare program has required hospitals and extended-care facilities to have utilization review plans. In 1972, Professional Standards Review Organizations (PSRO) were established to assess medical necessity and quality of services provided to participants in government health plans. Peer Review Organizations (PRO) replaced PSROs in 1984 when the Department of Health and Human Services entered into contracts with 54 review organizations. Activities of PROs are defined and described in scope-of-work statements issued by the Health Care Financing Administration (HCFA). PROs are primarily concerned with controlling utilization and monitoring quality of services received by Medicare beneficiaries under the Prospective Payment System

(PPS). They conduct preadmission, concurrent, and retrospective record reviews; scrutinize trends in individual facility admission, discharge, and transfer practices; and validate patient diagnosis related group (DRG) classifications. Legislation enacted in 1985 and 1986 expanded the scope of the PRO program to include reviews of services for Medicare beneficiaries in health maintenance organizations (HMOs) and competitive medical plans (CMPs), nursing facilities, and home health agencies.

Preferred provider organizations (PPOs) and health maintenance organizations (HMOs) attribute much of their success in controlling costs to strong utilization management. PPOs contract with providers who can demonstrate efficient service delivery practices and who will discourage inappropriate use of health-care services. Many PPOs require prior authorization for inpatient admissions or referral to specialists and mandate second surgical opinions for all elective surgical procedures. HMO's "gatekeeper" system places the primary-care professional in control of patients' access to services. For more information on utilization of services in PPOs and HMOs, see chapter 7 and Cornett (1987).

In their guide for hospital utilization review committees, Lamprey and Berry (1984) suggest that the term *utilization review* is outmoded and that *utilization management* more accurately reflects the current focus on prospective and concurrent control of resource allocation and utilization. The authors also describe one of the many computerized UR systems now available to assist reviewers in data collection, monitoring, and analysis. The purpose of Lamprey and Berry's system is to determine if the patient-care setting is appropriate for the services prescribed. The program is composed of screening criteria and review procedures. Criteria are of four types: (1) intensity of service, (2) appropriateness of service, (3) severity of illness, and (4) discharge screening. Criteria are applied to specific diagnoses, problems, and conditions for various body systems. Review procedures are included for admission, appropriateness, continued stay, and discharge. Although computer programs and systems vary, computerized utilization review or management activities much like the one discussed here are common in many health-care settings.

Risk Management

The goals of quality assurance and risk-management programs are very similar: prevent or identify and report errors early, resolve problems, and continue to monitor for possible deficiencies. The overall objective of both activities is to decrease adverse outcomes and increase desired outcomes, thereby enhancing the quality of care. For that reason, many health-care facilities include risk management in quality assurance programs. According to a report by the American Hospital Association (1987), the American Society of Health Care Risk Management defines risk management as

> An insurance and quality control related discipline comprising activities designed to minimize adverse effects of loss upon a health care organization's human, physical

and financial assets through: identification and assessment of loss potential; loss prevention and reduction; loss funding and risk financing; and professional, general liability, and workers' compensation claims control. (p. 9)

Risk-management personnel carry out a wide variety of activities, ranging from instituting safety and security procedures for staff, patients, and visitors to working with utilization review staff on developing admission and discharge criteria. Risk managers may also meet with professional and other facility staff to plan procedures for obtaining patient consent, ensuring confidentiality of medical records, and reporting incidents. Many hospitals now have computerized reporting systems that code incidents such as: patient choking, leave without consent, accidental injuries, medication errors, serious drug reactions, property damage, and episodes of physical or verbal abuse. Early and complete documentation of incidents assists risk managers in minimizing the health facility's liability exposure as well as in examining problem areas and identifying risks that can be corrected before loss is incurred.

The content and conduct of risk-management programs vary. Some facilities focus only on the safety and security aspects of risk, whereas others have a comprehensive quality assurance/utilization review/risk-management program. Even if the three activities are housed in separate departments or units, risk management can be considered a component of the overall quality-assurance program (Affeldt & Walczak, 1984).

QUALITY OF CARE IN SPEECH-LANGUAGE PATHOLOGY AND AUDIOLOGY

ASHA Standards Programs

Efforts to evaluate the quality of care in the speech-language pathology and audiology profession have evolved much like the attempts to assess quality in the wider health-care system. Initial efforts addressed the structural aspects of quality by developing standards for practitioner certification and program accreditation. Standards demonstrate to the public, regulatory agencies, and payors that the credentialed practitioner or accredited facility has or should have the capability to provide necessary, appropriate, and timely services (Flower, 1983).

The Council on Professional Standards in Speech-Language Pathology and Audiology (Standards Council) defines standards for clinical certification as well as accreditation of professional services programs and institutions that offer graduate education in speech-language pathology and audiology. Standards are interpreted and applied by three entities that comprise the Boards of Examiners in Speech-Language Pathology and Audiology (BESPA): Clinical Certification Board (CCB), Educational Standards Board (ESB), and the Professional Services Board (PSB).

Standards for Accreditation of Professional Services Programs

The purposes of the voluntary Professional Services Board (PSB) accreditation program, established in 1961, are to (1) encourage effective clinic management and high-quality services, (2) assure the best possible service to the public, and (3) provide a nationally recognized accreditation mechanism for professional clinical service programs in speech-language pathology and audiology. Through a rigorous application and site-visit process, PSB evaluates clinic programs and awards accreditation to those programs that are able to comply with all of its 25 standards. Accreditation is for a five-year period, subject to annual review by PSB. Standards are set for the following areas of review:

- Program goals
- Administration
- Services
- Personnel
- Records
- Physical plant and equipment
- Program evaluation/quality assurance

Standard 25, "Program Evaluation and Quality Assurance," is reprinted here because it is of particular interest in this chapter.

> The program shall evaluate the efficiency and effectiveness of the various components of its operations, including personnel, budget, equipment, facilities, and needs of the population served. This evaluation shall be accomplished by means of regular reviews of these components. Such reviews shall include formal evaluation of individual client management. (p. 15)

A complete description of standards and the accreditation process is provided in the PSB *Accreditation Manual*.

Standards for the Certificates of Clinical Competence

According to ASHA's "Requirements for the Certificates of Clinical Competence" in the *Membership and Certification Handbook* (1986), the Certificate of Clinical Competence (CCC-SLP and/or CCC-A) are awarded to "individuals who present satisfactory evidence of their ability to provide independent clinical services to persons who have disorders of communication" (p. 1). In addition to holding a master's degree or its equivalent with major emphasis in speech-language pathology, audiology, or speech-language and hearing science, the individual must meet specific standards with respect to general background education, required education, academic clinical practicum, completion of the Clinical Fellowship Year (CFY), and satisfactory performance on either (or both) of the National Examinations in Speech-Language Pathology and Audiology. Readers should refer to ASHA's *Membership and Certification Handbook* for specific requirements and information about the application process. In states that require licensure for the independent practice of speech-language pathology or audiology, individuals should contact the appropriate state licensing agency for information about requirements and application processes. Information is also available by contacting ASHA's State and Regulatory Policy Division in the Governmental Affairs Department.

Standards for Accreditation of Educational Institutions

The Educational Standards Board establishes criteria for approval of professional education (master's degree) programs and publicly identifies those programs that maintain adequate standards. Institutions seeking accreditation must complete a formal evaluation process that includes application, initial evaluation, site visit, and ESB review and approval (or disapproval) of application. Accreditation is awarded for a five-year period to programs that comply with its requirements. Annual reports must be submitted to the ESB for review. Standards have been established for the following aspects of the educational program:

- Program self-analysis
- Administration
- Curriculum
- Clinical practicum
- Faculty
- Institutional policy
- Facilities

Readers are directed to the Educational Standards Board publication *Accreditation of Educational Programs in Speech-Language Pathology and Audiology* (1984) for specific information.

Quality Assessment in Speech-Language Pathology and Audiology

In 1976, ASHA began to develop formal peer-review procedures for use in health-care and educational settings. The first system, the Patient Care Audit, was described by Griffin (1976) and Adair and Griffin (1979). ASHA's workshop manual, titled *Quality Assurance through Patient Care Audit*, was published in 1978. Another workshop manual, *Multidisciplinary Quality Review* (ASHA, 1978), was designed for advanced patient-care auditing procedures using group techniques. The *Child Services Review System* (ASHA, 1982) is a modification of the Patient Care Audit for use in speech-language-hearing or special education programs to assess and improve the effectiveness of services provided to handicapped students.

The Patient Care Audit system uses a team approach to evaluating and improving patient care on a continuous basis. Predetermined, objective criteria are developed by the professionals whose care is being reviewed for the purpose of identifying and correcting discrepancies between established criteria and standards of care and actual care provided. Superior evaluation and treatment procedures and patient outcomes may also be identified by this process. Services provided to individual patients by a specific speech-language pathologist or audiologist are not the focus of the retrospective review procedures. Rather, the purposes is to identify patterns of service delivery among clinicians in a given practice setting so that future patient care may be improved.

The Patient Care Audit system uses either process or outcome criteria to assess the critical indicators of care. Outcome criteria refer to the status of a patient following diagnosis and/or specific periods of treatment; process criteria evaluate aspects of patient care such as appropriateness of treatment objectives, essential components of diagnostic evaluations, or elements of discharge plans. All criteria must meet five necessary characteristics, commonly represented by the acronym RUMBA: relevant, understandable, measurable, behavioral, and achievable. Criteria are incorporated into seven sequential steps of the audit process. These steps are based upon the QA Loop procedure used in the health-care system (see Figure 8.2). ASHA's Patient Care Audit sequence follows:

1. Select audit topic (area of patient care);
   —Specify audit objective (purpose for audit—assess, evaluate, improve a specific aspect of patient care);
2. Draft criteria (professionals list critical indicators of quality care);
3. Ratify criteria (all professionals whose care is being audited agree on critical indicators);
4. Review patient charts:
5. Identify problems;
6. Analyze problems;
7. Develop solutions;
8. Implement solutions;
9. Reaudit.

Readers are referred to the manual *Quality Assurance through Patient Care Audit* for specific information on all aspects of completing a retrospective peer-review procedure.

Frattali (1986) updated procedures for evaluating quality in speech-language pathology by focusing her work on outcome assessment, incorporating mechanisms for prospective and concurrent reviews as well as the traditional retrospective methods. Interviews, surveys, the computer, or other data sources may be used in addition to, or in place of, the patient record. She offers an outcome-assessment protocol based on the work of Donabedian (1980) and Greeley and Stearns (1984). This protocol is presented in Figure 8.3.

Given the lack of empirically based criteria for assessing patient outcomes as well as the difficulty presented by attempts to account for intervening patient variables, Frattali does not advocate the use of outcome assessment without considering treatment processes. The importance of relating process and outcome variables in evaluating speech-language pathology and audiology services was

FIGURE 8.3
Outcome-Assessment Protocol

1. Select a disorder for study.
2. Define the patient population.
   Patient population is usually defined by diagnosis, age group, sex, severity of disorder, etc. The group should be homogeneous in order to limit possible intervening variables.
3. Determine an outcome topic.
   Topic may include such elements as: functional communication level, articulation accuracy, patient satisfaction, goal attainment, adjustment to hearing aids, etc.
4. Set a time frame to monitor.
   For example, if measuring esophageal speech proficiency, a time frame of six months post-operatively might be set.
5. Choose a method of assessment.
   Prospective
   Concurrent
   Retrospective
6. Select a data source.
   Data source is typically clinical record review, interview, survey, observation, or questionnaire.
7. Develop criteria for quality care for outcome elements.
   This is the most critical aspect of the evaluation. Explicit criteria, based on empirical research findings, are preferred.
8. Set the standards of care.
   Standards of care are usually designated by a percentage. If a 100 percent standard is set for the criterion, then 100 percent of all cases reviewed must satisfy the criterion to conclude that quality care has been provided.
9. Indicate acceptable exceptions to criteria.
   There are always cases in which nonconformance with criteria and standards is justified. For example, criteria may not be met because the patient demonstrated poor compliance, frequently cancelled treatment sessions, has certain physical or emotional complications, etc.
10. Provide explicit instructions for data collection.
11. Collect the data.
    Measure actual patient care using criteria and standards.
12. Analyze and summarize findings.
13. Interpret results.
14. Formulate corrective action to correct any deficiencies found.
15. Monitor care provided until deficiencies are corrected.

NOTE: Adapted from ''Are We Reaching Our Goals? Developing Outcome Measures'' by C. Frattali, May 1986, in P. Larkins (Ed.), *In Search of Quality Assurance: What Lies Ahead?* [ASHA Quality Assurance Workshop Manual]. Rockville, MD: ASHA. Adapted by permission.

also addressed by Adair and Griffin (1979). Donabedian (cited in Adair & Griffin, 1979) offers succinct advice for directing our efforts in this area:

> It is true that process elements can be used as indicators of quality only if there is a valid relation between these elements and desired outcomes. It is equally true that specific outcomes can be used as indicators of quality of care only to the extent that there is a valid relation between the two. Thus, validity resides not in the choice developments of process or outcomes but in what is known about their relationship. If a valid relation exists, either may be used, depending upon which can be more easily and accurately measured; if not, neither can be used. (pp. 857–858)

The task of relating treatment processes to outcomes was addressed by Vetter (1985), who suggested several procedures for evaluating clinical intervention, including establishing single or multiple baselines of client behaviors and attitudes, conducting pretest/post-test measures, and using a multiple target technique. She defined the multiple target technique as a successive series of pretest/post-test procedures in which only one behavior is treated while several behaviors are being observed. When the criterion is reached on the treated behavior, a different intervention is applied to the second behavior. At the same time, the clinician continues to measure other behaviors. According to Vetter, "When an adequate and stable baseline of behavior has been recorded and a treatment program instituted, changes in the behavior of interest allow the clinician to generate the hypothesis that the treatment resulted in the behavior change" (p. 63). She points out that replication of studies using similar clients and communication disorders is important in order to substantiate clinical findings.

Clinical research capabilities and needs have been the focus of considerable interest among other clinicians and researchers as well (e.g., Diggs, 1983; Frattali, 1986; Kent & Fair, 1985; McReynolds, 1983; Ringel, 1972; Siegel & Spradlin, 1985; Silverman, 1984). Silverman proposed that clinicians use a series of questions as a guide in determining the impact of treatment on patient outcomes. These questions first appeared in 1977 as components of Silverman's approach to assessing systematically the impacts of therapy methods in speech-language pathology and audiology on particular subpopulations of persons with communicative disorders.

- What are the effects of the therapy upon specific behaviors contributing to the client's communication disorder?
- What are the effects of therapy upon other attributes of a client's communication behavior? (side effects)
- What other effects is the therapy having upon the client?
- What are the client's attitudes toward the therapy and its effects upon his communicative and other behavior?
- What investment is required of client and clinician?
- What is the probability of relapse following termination of therapy? (1984, pp. 256–257)

According to Silverman (1984), the questions we ask ourselves in designing evaluation studies should be directly related to improving clinical effectiveness, and we should be able to establish easily a scientific rationale for answering them. Finally, it is perhaps Douglass's simply stated but complex question that best reflects one of our most pressing challenges today: "How do we know, and how can we show, that what we do in therapy really makes a difference?" (1983, p. 117).

New Directions in Evaluating the Quality of Care

The speech-language pathology and audiology profession is preparing for a new decade of clinical practice as methods are adapted or new techniques are developed for evaluating and improving the quality of services provided to communicatively impaired persons. In evaluating treatment processes and patient outcomes, practitioners will probably rely heavily on computers for data storage, retrieval, and analysis. Prospective and concurrent review criteria will be established according to regional and/or national standards and empirical research findings. The health-care consumer will also be an important source of data as the health-care system recognizes the influence of patient satisfaction and compliance on health outcomes. (See Chapey, 1977, and Adair & Griffin, 1979, for information on patient satisfaction as it relates to speech-language pathology and audiology services.) Finally, health-care professionals will work very closely with organizations and agencies such as the Joint Commission on Accreditation of Healthcare Organizations, insurance companies, employers, and Peer Review Organizations (PROs), all of which have developed or are currently initiating specific criteria for assessing quality and appropriate utilization of services for particular populations or practice settings.

The speech-language pathology and audiology profession is rapidly advancing in its efforts to respond to the challenges of evaluating quality of services with the development of new programs and procedures related to quality assurance, utilization review, and program evaluation.

Quality-Assurance and Utilization-Review Programs

ASHA's Committee on Quality Assurance, established in 1975, and the Professional Practices Division of the ASHA National Office have published or are developing a number of guides, statements, and reports related to quality-assurance and utilization-review activities in speech-language pathology and audiology. The *QA Digest* series is designed to keep members of the association informed about trends in various aspects of evaluating quality of care. Individual *Digests* are available on the following topics:

> Quality Assurance
> Quality Assurance and Utilization Review
> Outcome Assessment: An Overview

Program Evaluation
Performance Appraisal
Single-Subject Research Designs
Infection Control
Joint Commission on Accreditation of Healthcare Organizations
    (Standards for Rehabilitation Services)

ASHA's *QA Digest* on "Quality Assurance and Utilization Review" (Larkins, 1986) serves to illustrate the application of utilization-review and management activities used in the wider health-care system to speech-language pathology and audiology services. Larkins's recommendations for establishing utilization-review programs are summarized in Figure 8.4.

A second ASHA project involved the development of quality indicators that address the process component of quality assessment. The Committee on Quality Assurance prepared the report "Quality Assurance Process Indicators" (1987) which can be used by speech-language pathologists and audiologists in evaluating and monitoring services. Specific quality indicators are described for diagnostic and treatment procedures. There is also a list of generic indicators that apply to both areas. Some examples of diagnostic data that should be documented are patient's level of functional independence; hearing status; language skills; cognitive status; cranial, facial, and pharyngeal structure and function; and prognosis for rehabilitation of communication skills. Treatment indicators include the presence of treatment and discharge plans, descriptions of specific treatment approaches and techniques used, and ongoing assessment data. These indicators can be used to monitor and evaluate speech-language pathology and audiology services in any practice setting for all communication disorders. The committee is planning to prepare a report that will address disorder-specific process indicators. The committee's work is consistent with the health-care community's focus on developing common criteria and national data bases of quality and utilization information applicable to all practitioners in a given profession.

Additional ASHA projects on quality of care and utilization review in preparation include (1) a manual on staff-performance appraisal; (2) an educational program on conducting concurrent reviews; and (3) guidelines on developing review criteria for use by both state speech-language-hearing associations and speech-language pathology and audiology consultants to Medicare fiscal intermediaries and other third-party payors. The new Program Evaluation System (PES), however, is ASHA's major contribution to evaluating and monitoring quality of care in speech-language pathology and audiology programs.

ASHA's Program Evaluation System

The Program Evaluation System (PES) is an automated, multipurpose program-management system. Using the computer as its data source, the PES provides a mechanism for demonstrating attainment of program objectives and documenting

FIGURE 8.4
Utilization of Speech-Language Pathology and Audiology Services

Prospective, Concurrent, and Retrospective Utilization-Review Activities
Establish criteria for:

1. Necessity of admission-to-treatment program
2. Frequency of treatment
3. Intensity of treatment
4. Length of stay
5. Discharge

Determining Length of Stay (LOS):

1. Establish a data base of information on average length of treatment for patients in the program. Consider the following variables:
   Type of communication disorder
   Severity level
   Level of functional independence
   Type, frequency, and intensity of treatment
   Patient's age, sex, educational level
2. Compare average length of stay with that of other similar facilities and patient populations. Also review research findings.

Determining Timeliness and Appropriate Use of Services:

1. Compare date patient was initially seen by referral source and date patient was referred to SLP/A program.
2. Review date between initial SLP/A visit/diagnostic session and date treatment began.
3. Compare date patient was referred by SLP/A to another professional and date SLP/A received report or other information.
4. Review number and types of referrals from all sources to detect patterns of under- or over-utilization of services.

Conduct Staff Productivity Studies:

1. How many patients are seen by each clinician per day/week/month?
2. How are schedules determined?
3. What is the turnaround time for writing patient reports?
4. How is time allotted for staff development, clinical research, and other related activities?

Use Quality Assurance Procedures to Assess Utilization Data

1. Identify specific utilization problems.
2. Evaluate identified problems.
3. Report findings.
4. Develop an action plan to resolve problems.
5. Conduct follow-up studies to determine if problems are resolved.
6. Continue monitoring utilization data.

treatment processes and patient outcomes. Prospective, concurrent, and retrospective reviews may be conducted to assess and monitor the quality of speech-language pathology and audiology services and programs in all practice settings.

Six major files are included in the main-menu program structure:

1. Client Admission Data
2. Client Program Data
   (referral, assessment, schedule, procedure, attendance information)
3. Client Plan/Discharge Data
   (assessment and treatment protocols, discharge and follow-up plans, client peer review)
4. Staff Information
   (qualifications, continuing education, supervision, salaries, staff peer review)
5. Reports
   (client and program)
6. Utilities
   (site-specific administration and program peer-review data)

Four code lists are included with the "reports" menu. They are:

1. The ASHA Classification of Speech-Language Pathology and Audiology Procedures and Communication Disorders;
2. Functional communication measures (FCMs) for all communication systems;
3. Severity rating scales;
4. General codes.

The system generates 14 generic reports and, as a relational data base, has the capacity to produce more than 150 customized reports, according to user and program or facility needs. PES follows clients from program entry through discharge and follow-up. Functional status, communication diagnosis, and severity rating can be tracked throughout the treatment process to chart progress, monitor and adjust length of treatment, and document outcomes. Administrative uses of the PES include tracking payment sources and referral patterns, monitoring caseload size, determining fees per procedure, and storing demographic data on program staff and clients. PES permits uniform data collection while also ensuring confidentiality of information.

Users also have the opportunity to participate in establishing a national data base of information related to structure, process, and outcome variables in clinical practice. The data base will allow the profession to generate extensive utilization data, study severity levels and functional communication status across the spectrum of communication disorders, and track outcomes across practice settings.

The development of PES puts the speech-language pathology and audiology profession at the forefront of the health-care community's efforts to document treatment effectiveness and program efficiency. According to Larkins (1987),

PES allows the user to demonstrate efficient use of resources, maintain accountability, improve the quality of services provided, provide data necessary for planning and decision-making, demonstrate client outcomes, and improve public relations. PES is ASHA's tool to provide our data and not our word that speech-language pathologists and audiologists are providing quality speech-language-hearing services. (p. 24)

■ SUMMARY

Responding to increasing demands for quality and value in delivery of services, the health-care community has begun to develop and refine the concept of quality as well as methods to evaluate patient-care and health-care programs. Quality-assurance programs have been expanded to include utilization review and risk management as further evidence that quality of care is influenced and enhanced by a broad spectrum of activities. Providers will continue to be challenged in their efforts to establish empirically based criteria for evaluating their services. Although frustrations will accompany these efforts, both professionals and patients should benefit from the results. Quality has become the central issue in health care today.

The speech-language pathology and audiology profession's commitment to providing the best possible services to persons with communication disorders is reflected in its attention to all three approaches to quality assessment—structure, process, and outcome. ASHA's standards for individual practitioners, educational programs, and professional services have long provided a structural base for assuring professional excellence. More recently, the association's educational efforts and publications have been directed toward evaluating and improving treatment processes and patient/client outcomes. At the same time, the profession is in the midst of examination and debate about the complex interactions between research and clinical practice. Clinical research will likely play a much greater role in the everyday practice of speech-language pathologists and audiologists in the future. Finally, the profession will be well equipped to meet the new challenges of the next decade with its Program Evaluation System. This system represents state-of-the-are technology and evaluation techniques. Speech-language pathology and audiology is a profession in transition. We are poised to enter a new era of accountability, assisted by technology but guided by our principles, ethics, and dedication to those we serve.

ACTIVITIES

1. Invite the clinic director of the university clinic (or other program) to a class session to discuss the clinic's quality-assurance program.

2. Visit a clinic or speech-language-hearing program in a setting in which you would like to practice. Interview the director and/or staff members. You might ask the following questions:
   a. How is quality of care assessed?
   b. Is there a quality assurance program?

    c. What are the requirements for staff qualifications and job performance? Is there a staff development program?

    d. How does the speech-language-hearing program comply with facility wide requirements for quality assurance (if applicable)?

    e. How is the decision made to discharge a patient?

    f. Is the clinic or program currently conducting any program-evaluation studies or other clinic research? If not, are there plans for such studies?

The interviewer can determine other questions.

3. If possible, conduct a quality review using the "Outcome Assessment Protocol" (Figure 8.3). This would be an appropriate group project. Patient confidentiality must be assured. If it is not possible to use existing cases in the clinic, a retrospective review using the records of patients who have been discharged may be possible.

4. Develop one or more of the following for a hypothetical speech-language-hearing program (not for individual patients):

    a. Guidelines for discharge planning

    b. Clinic follow-up protocol

    c. Program-evaluation research proposal

    d. Guidelines for termination of treatment

    e. Patient satisfaction survey

    f. Staff development program

    g. Continuing education seminar on quality of care

    h. Guidelines for diagnostic assessments

    i. Guidelines for development of treatment plans

5. Prepare an annotated bibliography of quality-assessment, quality-assurance, or program-evaluation literature in a field other than speech-language pathology and audiology (e.g., physical therapy, psychology, social work, medicine). How does this information compare with the available literature and programs in speech-language pathology and audiology? What unique problems do other professions face in attempting to evaluate and quantify their services?

6. Write a position paper on evaluating the quality of care in speech-language pathology and audiology.

REFERENCES

Adair, M., & Griffin, K. (1979). Quality assurance: A professional quest for speech-language pathologists and audiologists. *Asha, 21*(10), 871–874.

Affeldt, J., & Walczak, R. (1984). The role of JCAH in assuring quality care. In J. Pena et al. (Eds.), *Hospital quality assurance* (pp. 49–62). Rockville, MD: Aspen.

American Hospital Association. (1987). *Managing risks and quality in hospital-sponsored home care.* Chicago, IL: Hospital Research and Educational Trust.

Arnold, W., & Leonard, M. (1987). HMOs and PPOs: An operational guide. *Topics in Health Care Financing, 13*(3), 19–31.

ASHA. (1982). *Child services review system manual.* Rockville, MD: ASHA.

ASHA. (1987). *Program evaluation system operations manual.* Rockville, MD: ASHA.

ASHA. (1978). *Quality assurance through patient care audit.* Rockville, MD: ASHA.

ASHA Clinical Certification Board (1986, June). *Membership and certification handbook.* Rockville, MD: ASHA.

ASHA Committee on Quality Assurance (1987). *Quality assurance process indicators.* Rockville, MD: ASHA.

ASHA Educational Standards Board (1984). *Accreditation of educational programs in speech-language pathology and audiology.* Rockville, MD: ASHA.

ASHA Professional Services Board (1984). *Accreditation manual.* Rockville, MD: ASHA.

Chapey, R. (1977). Consumer satisfaction in speech-language pathology. *Asha, 19*(1), 829–833.

Cornett, B. (1987). Managed care: A primer. *Governmental Affairs Review, 8*(1), 38–42.

Diggs, C. (1983). Professional accountability: Present and future directions. *Seminars in Speech and Language, 4*(2), 169–185.

Donabedian, A. (1969). *A guide to medical care administration, II: Medical care appraisal—Quality and utilization.* Washington, DC: American Public Health Association.

———. (1978). The quality of medical care. *Science, 200,* 856–864.

———. (1980). *The definition of quality and approaches to its assessment.* Ann Arbor, MI: Health Administration Press.

Donabedian, A., Wheeler, J., & Wyszewianski, L. (1984). An integrative model of quality, cost, and health. In J. Pena et al. (Eds.), *Hospital quality assurance* (pp. 65–88). Rockville, MD: Aspen.

Douglass, R. (1983). Defining and describing clinical accountability. *Seminars in Speech and Language, 4*(2), 107–118.

Flower, R. (1983). Professional standards and accountability. *Seminars in Speech and Language, 6*(1), 119–129.

———. (1984). *Delivery of speech-language pathology and audiology services.* Baltimore, MD: Williams & Wilkins.

Frattali, C. (1986, May). Are we reaching our goals? Developing outcome measures. In P. Larkins (Ed.), *In search of quality assurance: What lies ahead?* [ASHA Quality Assurance Workshop Manual]. Rockville, MD: ASHA.

Greeley, H., & Stearns, G. (1984, December). Primer on retrospective outcome audit. *Quality Review Bulletin,* 438–441.

Griffin, K. (1976). Quality assurance through patient care audit. *Asha, 18*(11), 800–803.

———. (1978). *Multidisciplinary quality review: Advanced patient care audit workshop manual.* Rockville, MD: ASHA.

Haffner, A., Jonas, S., & Pollack, B. (1984). Regulating the quality of patient care. In J. Pena et al. (Eds.), *Hospital quality assurance* (pp. 3–24). Rockville, MD: Aspen.

Health Standards and Quality Bureau, Health Care Financing Administration, Department of Health, Education and Welfare (1978). *Handbook for conduct of medical care evaluation studies.* Washington, DC: U.S. Government Printing Office.

Joint Commission on Accreditation of Hospitals (1986). *Accreditation manual for hospitals/87.* Chicago, IL: JCAH.

Kearns, P. (1984). Quality assurance and utilization review. In J. Pena et al. (Eds.), *Hospital quality assurance* (pp. 237–252). Rockville, MD: Aspen.

Kent, R., & Fair, J. (1985). Clinical research: Who, where, and how? *Seminars in Speech and Language, 6*(1), 23–24.

Lamprey, J., & Berry, N. (1984). *A guide to utilization management.* Chicago, IL: InterQual, Inc.

Larkins, P. (1986). Quality assurance and utilization review. *Quality Assurance Digest.* Rockville, MD: ASHA.

———. (1987). Program evaluation system (PES): Determining quality of speech-language-hearing services. *Asha, 29*(5), 21–26.

McReynolds, L. (1983). Discussion: Part VII: Evaluating program effectiveness. In J. Miller, D. Yoder, and R. Schiefelbusch (Eds.), *Contemporary issues in language intervention* (pp. 298–306). Rockville, MD: ASHA.

Pena, J., Rosen, B., Haffner, A., & Light, D. (Eds.) (1984). *Hospital quality assurance.* Rockville, MD: Aspen.

Ricci, E. (1985, Winter). Lecture notes for graduate course in evaluation research. Pittsburgh, PA: Graduate School of Public Health, University of Pittsburgh.

Ringel, R. (1972). The clinician and the researcher: An artificial dichotomy. *Asha, 14*(7), 351–353.

Siegel, G., & Spradlin, J. (1985). Therapy and research. *Journal of Speech and Hearing Disorders, 50*(3), 226–229.

Silverman, F. (1977). Criteria for assessing therapy outcome in speech pathology and audiology. *Journal of Speech and Hearing Research, 20*(1), 5–20.

———. (1984). *Speech-language pathology and audiology: An introduction.* Columbus, OH: Merrill.

Suchman, E. (1967). *Evaluative research.* NY: Russell Sage Foundation.

U.S. Congress, Office of Technology Assessment. (1986). *Payment for physicians' services: Strategies for Medicare.* OTA–H–294. Washington, DC: U.S. Government Printing Office.

Vetter, D. (1985). Evaluation of clinical intervention: Accountability. *Seminars in Speech and Language, 6*(1), 55–66.

EPILOGUE: CLINICAL PRACTICE IN THE NEXT DECADE

We have presented a comprehensive overview of clinical practice in speech-language pathology today. Our discussion has encompassed the many areas of knowledge with which a competent practitioner must be familiar. Today's theories and practices, however, quickly become obsolete as each of the aspects of professional practice evolves with changes in the health-care and educational systems. Thus, we must look into the future to anticipate trends and to prepare ourselves for the next decade and beyond. What will clinical practice be like in the year 2000?

If we surveyed 10 experienced speech-language pathologists and asked them to predict the status of clinical practice in 10 years, their answers would probably reflect their own clinical specialties and practice settings. Our field is composed of professionals whose interests are diverse and whose goals may sometimes be in conflict with those of their colleagues. Industrywide consensus is difficult to determine, but we will attempt to make some projections.

Clinical practice will likely be influenced by four major trends: (1) changing demographics, (2) the health-care system's focus on cost-effectiveness and quality assessment, (3) the changing role of allied health professionals within the system, and (4) the continuing evolution of technology (Larkins, 1986). As the population grows older, the need for services to the elderly will increase. By the year 2000, 25% of persons over age 65 are expected to have a speech or language impairment, and 46% may have a hearing impairment. Speech-language pathologists and audiologists will need to expand and improve service delivery components for this population. Clinical services will also be adapted to meet the needs of deinstitutionalized persons as well as minorities and a growing multicultural population. Additionally, services to infants and preschool children are increasing because of passage of recent legislation. New ways to deliver services to families in which both parents work full-time and the children are placed in day-care centers will also be developed.

The growing use of computers and other technologies in diagnosis, treatment, clinical administration, report writing, and research is exciting. The amount of sophisticated software available continues to increase rapidly. Articles, books, software reviews, and seminars on all phases of technology and clinical practice ensure that clinicians can keep pace with new developments and avail themselves of tools to enhance all phases of clinical practice.

The roles of nonphysician health-care professionals will undergo close scrutiny as administrators search for ways to use health-care personnel more efficiently. The demand for generalist or multiskilled practitioners and those who have enhanced their abilities through additional education and training is growing. Speech-language pathologists and audiologists will need to examine and reevaluate education, training, certification, and scope-of-practice requirements to determine where the profession might fit within that trend. The concept of specialty recognition and other continuing education opportunities are being further developed by ASHA.

Quality, cost-effectiveness, and efficiency are the key words in health care for at least the next decade. As a result, speech-language pathology and audiology services will be subjected to various types of quality assessment and utilization-review structures. Although this trend may be somewhat threatening at first glance, the profession's participation in developing guidelines and mechanisms for peer review will likely be a very positive force for clinical practice. A mature profession is one that sets its own carefully developed program for ensuring accountability among its members. ASHA's new Program Evaluation System (PES) is a very promising tool for developing a national data base of information on numerous variables related to quality, cost-effectiveness, and efficiency. In addition, ASHA has recently developed a classification system for professional procedures and communication disorders. This system establishes standard terminology and procedural definitions for the profession and will be an invaluable tool for research, reimbursement, and quality-assurance purposes.

ASHA's 1987 president, Patricia Cole, recently shared her observations and opnions about the future of the profession of speech-language pathology and audiology. Cole (1986) suggested that the profession has set the overall goal of moving from a supportive role to a primary role in the health-services delivery system, and she outlined the characteristics of a "primary profession" as follows:

1. Services provided are recognized widely as addressing an area of human functioning critical to well-being. These services are treated as essential components in the health services delivery system.
2. Members of the profession are recognized as experts in the area of human functioning for which they deliver services. They are primarily responsible for decisions concerning diagnosis and treatment of disorders in their area of expertise.
3. The profession accepts responsibility both for producing and applying new information in its own area of practice. It has a strong research component as well as a strong service delivery component.
4. The professionals are held directly accountable for the accuracy of their diagnoses and the effectiveness of their treatment programs.
5. The professionals are required by law to be licensed to practice. Standards for licensing and for ethical conduct are set and administered by the profession.
6. Services typically are covered in third-party reimbursement programs, both public and private.
7. The profession has both generalists and specialists. All have a basic, broad-based core of knowledge and skills that undergird more advanced specialization. (p. 41)

Cole contends that meeting these characteristics will require some changes for speech-language pathology and audiology education, training, and practices. She challenges the profession to raise the education and training requirements beyond two years of graduate study, to encourage advanced preparations and specializations, and to promote strong clinical research studies. Cole also believes that we must be more assertive in defining our roles and in publicizing our services and skills to the public as well as other professionals.

It will be interesting to review Cole's list in 5 years and again in 10 years. The result will probably be encouraging, as our profession now gives every indication that we have a promising future. Many of our parents have told us that "life is what you make it." The same is true for our profession. It will only advance as far as each of us is willing to take it. Will we be a primary profession in 10 years? The answer lies with you and me.

REFERENCES AND BIBLIOGRAPHY

REFERENCES

Cole, P. (1986). I want to shape my own future: How about you? *Asha, 28*(9), 41–42.
Larkins, P. (1986). The challenges ahead for the practice of speech-language pathology. *Asha, 28*(9), 29–30.

BIBLIOGRAPHY

ASHA. (1986). The autonomy of speech-language pathology and audiology. *Asha, 28*(5), 53–57.
Kamara, C. (1986) ASHA's professional practices activities. *Asha, 28*(9), 25–28.
Minifie, F. (1983). ASHA is planning for the future. *Asha, 25*(5), 29–30.

Appendix A

BRIEF OVERVIEW OF AUDIOLOGY

Audiologists are specialists in the prevention, identification, and assessment of hearing loss and hearing disorders, and in the habilitation and rehabilitation of persons who have hearing impairments. Services may include the fitting and dispensing of hearing aids. Audiologists also conduct research related to normal hearing processes, hearing loss, and hearing disorders.

Some activities of the audiologist include:

- Using sophisticated equipment and procedures to measure hearing ability and identify the presence, type, and severity of hearing problems.
- Prescribing hearing aids and other assistive listening devices; providing orientation and follow-up care.
- Counseling patients, families, teachers, and other persons who need to understand the problems associated with hearing impairments.
- Developing hearing-conservation programs in industry and the armed services to prevent hearing loss resulting primarily from noise exposure.
- Instructing hearing-impaired patients in speech reading and auditory training activities.
- Conducting early identification programs by evaluating infants' hearing, especially those at high risk for hearing impairment.
- Monitoring the effectiveness of devices and treatments used for patient management.

Audiologists work in a variety of settings, including hospitals, rehabilitation centers, physicians' offices, schools, private practice, universities and colleges, community clinics, industry, and public health agencies. A very small number of audiologists work in nursing facilities and home-care agencies. According to Cherow (1986), the top four audiology practice settings are (1) general or community hospital, (2) private physician's office, (3) college or university, and (4) own office. (Refer to the list of Recent Articles on Audiology in this appendix.) The majority of audiologists provides direct clinical services, but many are also engaged in administration, university teaching, consultation, supervision, and research. Survey data (Hyman, 1986a; 1986b) show that median basic annual salaries for audiologists in all practice settings are consistently higher than those of speech-language pathologists. For 1985 the median salary exceeded speech-language pathologist's median salary by almost $3,000.

The outlook for the practice of audiology appears to be very bright as audiologists increase the type and number of services they provide to expanded or new populations. The number of persons with hearing impairments is expected to increase at a rate 102% faster than the rate of growth of the total U.S. population between the years 1980 and 2050 as a direct result of the aging of the population (Fein, 1983). Consequently, more audiologists will be needed to serve these persons. In addition, audiologists are offering more prevention and hearing-conservation services; expanding their involvement with cochlear implants, vibrotactile devices, and interoperative monitoring; and dispensing hearing aids and other assistive devices. There is also a need to increase service delivery to institutionalized and multicultural populations. Clearly, the practice of audiology should present challenges and opportunities for many years to come.

RECENT ARTICLES ABOUT AUDIOLOGY

ASHA Ad Hoc Committee on Cochlear Implants. (1986). Report of the Ad Hoc Committee on Cochlear Implants. *Asha*, (4), 29–52.

ASHA Ad Hoc Committee on Extension of Audiology Services in the Schools. (1983). Audiology services in the schools. *Asha*, 25(5), 53–60.

ASHA Committee on Rehabilitative Audiology. (1984), Definition of and competencies for aural rehabilitation. *Asha*, 26, (5), 37–41.

ASHA Committee on Amplification for the Hearing Impaired. (1984). Guidelines for graduate training in amplification. *Asha*, 26(5), 43.

ASHA Staff. (1987). Dispensing quality: More than hearing aids are marketed in dispensing audiology practices. *Asha*, 29,(4), 22–27.

ASHA Task Force on the Definition of Hearing Handicap. (1981). On the definition of hearing handicap. *Asha*, 23(4), 293–297.

Cherow, E. (1986). The practice of audiology: A national perspective. *Asha*, 27(9), 31–38.

Fein, D. (1983). Projections of speech and hearing impairments to 2050. *Asha*, 25(11), 31.

Goldstein, D. (1984). Hearing impairment, hearing aids, and audiology. *Asha*, 26(9), 24–38.

Hyman, C. (1986a). 1985 ASHA omnibus survey. *Asha*, 28(4), 19–22.

Hyman, C. (1986b). More than a billion in earnings: An update on salaries in the speech-language-hearing profession. *Asha*, 28(7), 31–35.

Martin, F., & Sides, D. (1985). Survey of current audiometric practices. *Asha*, 27(2), 29–36.

Sullivan, C., & Sullivan, R. (1987). Hearing aid dispensing: Responsibilities, rewards, risks. *Asha*, 29(4), 37–40.

Wilson-Vlotman, A., & Blair, J. (1987). A survey of audiologists working full time in school systems. *Asha*, 28(11), 33–40.

Appendix B   Professional Journals, Associations, and Organizations

JOURNALS

Aging and Human Development
American Journal of Mental Deficiency
American Journal of Occupational Therapy
American Journal of Public Health
American Psychologist
Archives of Neurology
Archives of Otolaryngology
Archives of Physical Medicine and Rehabilitation
Audiology and Hearing Education
Behavioral Disorders
Brain
Brain and Language
Child Development
Cognitive Psychology
Congressional Quarterly
Cortex
Counseling Psychology
Dental Hygiene
Developmental Psychology
Dysphagia
Exceptional Children
Ear and Hearing

Geriatrics
Gerontology
Health Care Financing Review
Health Care Management Review
Health Education Quarterly
Health Policy Quarterly
Hearing Aid Journal
Hearing Instruments
Hospitals
International Journal of Rehabilitation
Journal of Abnormal Psychology
Journal of the Academy of Rehabilitative Audiology
Journal of Allied Health
Journal of Ambulatory Care Management
Journal of the American Medical Association
Journal of Autism and Developmental Disorders
Journal of Behavioral Assessment
Journal of Childhood Communication Disorders
Journal of Child Language
Journal of Communication Disorders
Journal of Computer Users in Speech-Language Pathology and Audiology (CUSH)
Journal of Educational Psychology
Journal of Experimental Child Psychology
Journal of Fluency Disorders
Journal of Health Politics, Policy and Law
Journal of Learning Disabilities
Journal of Pediatric Psychology
Journal of Psychoeducational Assessment
Journal of Verbal Larning and Verbal Behavior
Learning Disability Quarterly
Learning and Motivation
Mental Retardation
Milbank Memorial Fund Quarterly: Health and Society
Modern Healthcare
Neurology
Neuropsychologia
New England Journal of Medicine
Perspectives on Aging
Physical Therapy
Public Health Reports
Rehabilitation Literature
Rehabilitation World
Seminars in Speech and Language
Social Security Bulletin
Special Education
The Exceptional Parent
The Gerontologist
The Hearing Journal
The Lancet

The National Journal
Topics in Health Law
Topics in Language Disorders
Topics in Learning and Learning Disabilities
Volta Review

ASSOCIATIONS AND ORGANIZATIONS

Accrediting Commissions

Commission on Accreditation of Rehabilitation Facilities
2500 N. Patano Rd.
Tucson, AZ   85715

Joint Commission on Accreditation of Healthcare Organizations
875 N. Michigan Ave.
Chicago, IL   60611

Government Agencies

Health Care Financing Administration
6325 Security Blvd.
Baltimore, MD   21207
- Bureau of Eligibility, Reimbursement and Coverage
  (reimbursement policy)
- Health Standards and Quality Bureau
- Office of Prepaid Health Care
  (HMO contracting for Medicare beneficiaries)
- Bureau of Program Policy
  (coverage of services)
- Bureau of Program Operations
  (denials—Medicare claims)
- Office of Public Affairs

National Institute on Aging
Bldg. 31, Room 5035
NIH/NIA
900 Rockville Pike
Bethesda, MD   20205

National Institute of Child Health & Human Development
Landow Bldg., Room 7C03
NIH/NICHD
7910 Woodmont Ave.
Bethesda, MD   20205

National Institute of Neurological and Communicative Disorders and Stroke
Federal Bldg., Room 11C–11
NIH/NINCDS
7550 Wisconsin Ave.
Bethesda, MD   20205

National Science Foundation
Room 320
1800 G St., NW
Washington, DC   20550

Health Information

National Health Information Clearinghouse
P.O. Box 1135
Washington, DC   20013

National Rehabilitation Information Center
4407 Eighth St., NE
Washington, DC   20017

Interest Groups

Academy of Aphasia
c/o Antonio Damasio, MD
Dept. of Neurology
College of Medicine
University of Iowa
Iowa City, IA   52242

Alexander Graham Bell Association for the Deaf
3417 Volta Place, NW
Washington, DC   20007

Alzheimer's Disease and Related Disorders
360 N. Michigan Ave., Suite 1102
Chicago, IL   60601

American Association on Mental Deficiency (AAMD)
1719 Kalorama Rd., NW
Washington, DC   20009

American Cancer Society
90 Park Ave.
New York, NY   10016

American Cleft Palate Association
331 Salk Hall
University of Pittsburgh
Pittsburgh, PA   15261

American Foundation for the Blind
15 W. 16th St.
New York, NY   10011

American Parkinson Disease Association
116 John St., Suite 417
New York, NY   10038

Association for Children and Adults with Learning Disabilities (ACLD)
4156 Library Rd.
Pittsburgh, PA   15234

Council for Exceptional Children
1920 Association Drive
Reston, VA   22091

Gerontological Society of America
1411 K St., NW, Suite 300
Washington, DC   20005

March of Dimes Birth Defects Foundation
1275 Mamaroneck Ave.
White Plains, NY   10605

National Easter Seal Society for Crippled Children and Adults
2023 W. Ogden Ave.
Chicago, IL   60612

National Society for Children and Adults with Autism
1234 Massachusetts Ave., NW
Suite 1017
Washington, DC   20005

Professional Associations

American Affiliation of Visiting Nurse Associations and Services
21 Maryland Plaza, Suite 300
St. Louis, MO   63108

American Congress of Rehabilitation Medicine
30 N. Michigan Ave.
Chicago, IL   60602

American Dental Association
211 E. Chicago Ave.
Chicago, IL   60611

American Federation of Teachers
555 New Jersey Ave., NW
Washington, DC   20001

American Health Care Association
1200 15th St., NW
Washington, DC   20005

American Hospital Association
840 Lakeshore Drive
Chicago, IL   60611

American Medical Association
535 N. Dearborn St.
Chicago, IL   60610

American Nurses Association
2420 Pershing Road
Kansas City, MO   64108

American Occupational Therapy Association
1383 Piccard Dr.
Rockville, MD   20850

American Physical Therapy Association
1111 N. Fairfax St.
Alexandria, VA   22314

American Psychological Association
1200 17th St., NW
Washington, DC   20036

American Public Health Association
1015 15th St., NW
Washington, DC   20005

National Association for Home Care
519 C. Street, NE Stanton Park
Washington, DC   20002

National Association of Rehabilitation Facilities
P.O. Box 17675
Washington, DC   20041

National Association of Social Workers
7981 Eastern Ave.
Silver Spring, MD   20910

National Educational Association
1201 16th St., NW
Washington, DC   20036

National Rehabilitation Association
633 S. Washington St.
Alexandria, VA   22314

Registry for Interpreters for the Deaf
814 Thayer Ave.
Silver Spring, MD   20910

Appendix C   Publications and Resources for Private Practitioners

AVAILABLE FOR PURCHASE FROM ASHA:

Determining Costs of Speech, Language, and Hearing Services (1985)
Health Insurance Manual for Speech-language Pathologists and Audiologists (1984)
Marketing Speech, Language, and Hearing Services (1987) (4 cassettes)
Planning and Initiating a Private Practice in Speech-Language Pathology and Audiology (1985)
Program Evaluation System (1987) (software and manual)
Quality Assurance Through Patient Care Audit (1982)
Services in Home Health Settings (1987) (2 cassettes)
Users Systems for Evaluating and Reviewing Software (USERS); Users I: Screening and Evaluation (1987)

OTHER ARTICLES AND BOOKS

ASHA Committee on Private Practice. (1982). Questions and answers on private practice. *Asha*, 24(11), 953–954.

Flower, R. (1984). *Delivery of clinical services in speech-language pathology and audiology.* Baltimore, MD: Williams & Wilkins.

McLauchlin, R. (Ed.). (1986). *Speech-language pathology and audiology: Issues and management.* Orlanda, FL: Grune & Stratton.

Wood, M. (1986). *Private practice in communication disorders.* Boston, MA: College-Hill.

Appendix D   Long-Term-Care Resources

ASHA PUBLICATIONS

Breaking the Silence Barrier: An In-Service Program for Long-Term Care Facilities Staff (1985)
Communication Disorders and Aging Package—slides, cassette, leader's guide, participant's manual, monograph; sold separately or together (1985)
Communication Problems of the Older American (1979)
Gerontology and Communication Disorders (1985)
Organizations and Agencies in the Area of Aging (1980)
Resource Materials for Communication Problems of Older Persons (1980)

OTHER BOOKS AND ARTICLES

ASHA. (1980). Aging and communication: A special look. [Special issue]. *Asha, 22*(6).
Beasley, D., & Davis, G. (Eds.). (1981). *Aging: Communication processes and disorders.* New York: Grune & Stratton.
Fein, D. (1984). On aging. *Asha, 26*(8), 25.
Larkins, P. (1986). Serving the deinstitutionalized mentally retarded and developmentally disabled population: What are the issues? *Asha, 28*(11), 43–46.
Mueller, P., & Peters, T. (1981). Needs and services in geriatric speech-language pathology and audiology. *Asha, 23*(9), 627–632.
Nuru, N. (1985). Institutionalized people: Can we do a better job? *Asha, 27*(1), 35–38.
Oyer, H., & Oyer, E. (Eds.). (1976). *Aging and communication.* Baltimore, MD: University Park Press.
Ventry, I., & Weinstein, B. (1983). Identification of elderly people with hearing problems. *Asha, 25*(7), 37–42.

Appendix E Consent to Release Information*

TO: _____   RE: _____
              Agency   Client

_____   _____

_____   _____

The Speech and Hearing Clinic has been requested and authorized to forward to your agency the following information pertaining to the above-named client:

Title	*Date of Document*
1. _____	_____
2. _____	_____
3. _____	_____

Should you have any questions regarding the enclosed information, please feel free to contact our clinic.

_____ _____
Signature of Clinical Supervisor   Date

_____ _____
Signature of person authorized   Date
to consent for release of above
listed and enclosed information

_____
Relation to Client

*Appendices E through M from Division of Communication Disorders, Department of Communication, University of Pittsburgh. Used with permission.

Appendix F   Diagnostic Report Format

Speech and Language Diagnostic Report

Name: Date of Diagnostic:
Address: Informant for History:
Birth Date: Parents:
Sex: Referral Source:
Telephone: (Name, Address and Phone)

   I. *Complaint and Referral*   (Description of problem according to informant: how and why
                                did client seek service at this clinic.)

  II. *History*
      A. Family
      B. Developmental/Medical
      C. Speech and Language Development
      D. Social-Educational

 III. *Evaluation*
      A. Language
         1. Receptive (formal and informal results, clinical observation)
         2. Expressive (formal and informal results, clinical observation)
                language sample analysis
      B. Articulation (formal and informal results)
      C. Voice
      D. Fluency
      E. Oral Peripheral Examination
      F. Hearing Results of an audiological evaluation conducted by Audiology Super-
         visor, CCC-A indicated. . .
      G. Other Significant Factors (i.e., behavior, parent-child interaction)

 IV. Clinical Impressions and Diagnosis

  V. Recommendations (include preferred days/times for therapy)

_____   _____
Name, CCC-SLP   Name
Clinical Supervisor   Graduate Student Clinician

Appendix G   Flowchart Guidelines

Client _____   Date _____

Clinician _____   Session # _____

Problem #	Objectives	Procedures	Results
Amount of time alloted for activity (6 min.)	Short-term goal(s) written in behavioral terms including the following information: 1. What the client is expected to do 2. Under what conditions/circumstances 3. Criterion level based on percentage correct, specific number of correct responses, time limit, etc.	techniques, specific tasks, types of materials, method of reinforcement to be used to achieve goal(s)	Observable data recorded during session when applicable. Stimulus items listed prior to session.
Example #1	The client will spontaneously produce /s/[1] in monosyllabic words with 90% accuracy. (Please leave space between objectives for supervisor's comments.)	Peabody Picture Cards to serve as stimuli in rapid fire-drill; fixed ratio reinforcement schedule (after every 3 correct responses). Indicate number of stimulus items. Activity reinforcer following completion of activity—paint with water	
Example #2	The client will produce /+ ʃ/ in isolation following clinician's model with 16 out of 20 correct.	Auditory and visual cues; clinician serves as verbal model, phonetic placement cues; motivational activity of train going down track; sound of train associated with target phoneme, continuous reinforcement, sticker upon completion of task.	

Results for Example #1:

	Trials		
	1	2	3
sun	+	−	+
soup	−	+	+
sea	−	+	+
saw	+	+	−
soap	−	+	+
etc.	+	+	+

+ = correct
− = incorrect
/+ ʃ/

Appendix H Flowchart

Client _____ Clinician _____ Supervisor, CCC-SP _____ Term/Year _____

Problem Number	OBJECTIVE:	Date	ETA

Supervisor's Initials/Dates →

Therapy Variables

% CORRECT

100%
95%
90%
85%
80%
75%
70%
65%
60%
55%
50%

Appendix I   Progress-Notes Form

PROGRESS NOTES FOR _____

DATE	PROBLEM NUMBER	NOTE

Appendix J   Summary Progress Report

File Number

Name: Referral Source
Address: Name:
Birth Date: Address:
Sex: Date of Diagnostic:
Telephone: Period Covered by Summary:
School/Occupation: Date of Report:
Parents: Number of Sessions Scheduled:
                                             Number of Sessions Attended:
                                             Accumulative Sessions:

BACKGROUND INFORMATION

General introductory statements regarding nature and severity of client's primary problem; date and location of diagnostic, brief summary of results and recommendations, medical diagnosis (i.e., mental retardation); etiology, if known (structural, organic, or neurological); duration of past therapy; primary emphasis of previous therapy; description of progress made and recommendations; present vocational/education situation and living arrangement of client if new or important to case. If first-term client, more specific information regarding case history. Occasionally references to pertinent previous reports may be made. However, routine reference is not recommended. Schedule planned for term—frequency of sessions/group-individual/counseling.

THERAPY PROCESS

Status at onset of current therapy period, current objective(s), plan(s), and progress to date for each active problem.

Problem No. 1—*Short Title*

All relevant information from problem statement as known at beginning of current therapy period. Report documentation of problem from formal and informal test results, examinations, or reports from others. The problem statements do not contain exaggerated or unsupported conclusions. They do not include nonproblems; for example, Hearing—normal. The statements should be updated each term.

Objective(s)

Statement of criterion-referenced behavioral objective(s), time limited by end of therapy period.

Plan(s)

Description of therapy strategies including therapy model, types of materials/activities/procedures, reinforcement system, may include examples.

Progress

Objective results including response data, documentation of progress or lack thereof (post-testing comparison to pretesting).

Problem No. 2—*Short Title*

(Format for Problem 1, above, to be followed for all problems addressed.)

NOTE: This report must serve as a summary of flowcharts and progress notes.

CLINICAL IMPRESSIONS (Subjective Information)

How client and his/her parent/guardian/significant others view the progress of the therapy period.

Analysis of adequacy, appropriateness, and effectiveness of therapy. Relate objectives for term and client assessment to your assessment. If initial recommended objectives, plans and/or schedule were not carried out, an explanation must be provided. Current impression of overall speech/language status. Statement of prognosis for further or continued growth. Examples: In view of (state reasons, e.g., stimulability/motivation) overall prognosis for this client appears (e.g., favorable). Prognosis for continued growth for (skill) remains positive, however, prognosis for (skill) appears poor.

RECOMMENDATIONS

Begin with brief statement relating assessment of progress to recommendations. General plan to continue therapy (frequency, duration, type, group/individual, estimate of treatment period) discharge or transfer. Specific plan(s) or recommendations for next therapy period including diagnostic, referrals, follow-up, further client education, parent counseling, parent involvement with therapy process. Statement verifying that these recommendations were discussed with client and client's reaction to recommendation. Specific statements regarding future therapy emphasis (problem priorities). General therapy approach and tentative objectives.

(Written Signature)	(Written Signature)
Typed Name, Degree, CCC-SLP	Typed Name B.S. or B.A.
Clinical Supervisor	Graduate Student Clinician

NOTE: The certified audiologist must cosign all Summary Progress Reports written for hearing-impaired clients.

Appendix K   Referral Form

Date _____

TO: _____   RE: _____
       Physician's Name   Client's Name

_____   _____
          Address   Address

_____   _____

_____
                                     Date of Birth

As routine procedure we request that clients receiving voice therapy be seen for a laryngeal examination. The purpose for such is twofold:

1. that we may rule out medical contraindications for specific therapeutic procedures and/or techniques;
2. that we may have anatomical/physiological points for comparison of pre- and post-treatment phases.

The above-named client has indicated to us that you are the physician of choice and has given us permission to contact you. Please advise us concerning the results of your examination. You may record your results on the form found on the reverse of this letter.

Thank you for your time and for sharing this information with us.

_____
Clinical Supervisor, CCC/Sp

_____
Graduate Student Clinician

Appendix L Request For Information

Date _____

To _____
                    Agency

_____

_____

Please release the records specified below to the attention of

_____ , _____ .
            Name   Title

at the Speech and Hearing Clinic.

Client's Name _____ _____

Information being requested: _____

_____

_____

_____

_____

_____

Release of information is authorized below.

_____   _____   _____
Signature of person authorized   Date   Signature of person
to consent for release of above   requesting information
information

_____
Relation to client

Appendix M   Consent Form for Observation and Taping

Consent for Observation and Audio and Video Taping of Evaluation and Therapy Sessions

Client _____ Date of Birth _____

Parents _____

Address _____

In consideration of the educational function of the Speech and Hearing Clinic, I give consent that I (we) and my child may be observed for research or educational purposes while receiving services at this Clinic. It is understood that the staff, observers, and students will consider any information revealed during such examinations or demonstrations as privileged communication and will hold such information in confidence, except when authorized by me (us) to release it to appropriate medical, social, educational, health or other agencies.

I also consent that audio and video recordings may be made for client records and/ or for use in education and research. It is understood that in such cases tapes will not be identified by name.

This form has been fully explained to me (us) and I (we) certify that its contents are understood.

_____

(Parent's or Client's Signature)

_____

(Date)

Author Index

Subject Index